YO-CDK-323

NURSING PHOTOBOOK

Caring for Surgical Patients

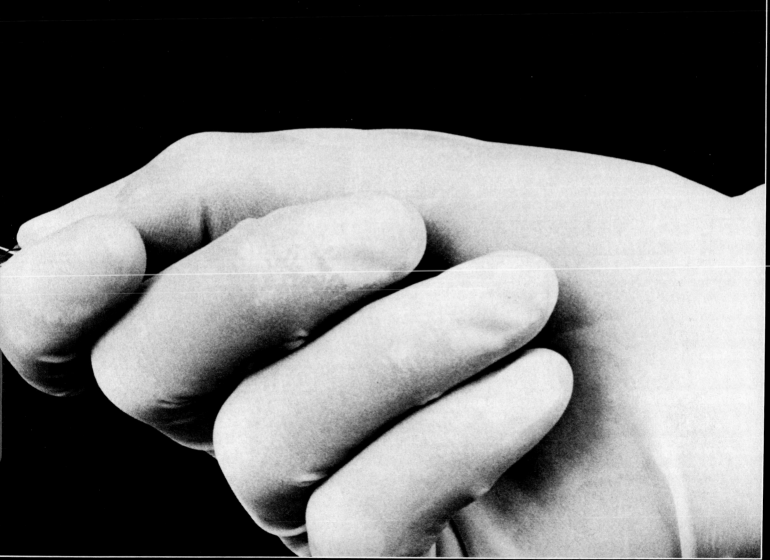

NURSING84 BOOKS™

NURSING PHOTOBOOK™ SERIES
Providing Respiratory Care
Managing I.V. Therapy
Dealing with Emergencies
Giving Medications
Assessing Your Patients
Using Monitors
Providing Early Mobility
Giving Cardiac Care
Performing GI Procedures
Implementing Urologic Procedures
Controlling Infection
Ensuring Intensive Care
Coping with Neurologic Disorders
Caring for Surgical Patients
Working with Orthopedic Patients
Nursing Pediatric Patients
Helping Geriatric Patients
Attending Ob/Gyn Patients
Aiding Ambulatory Patients
Carrying Out Special Procedures

NEW NURSING SKILLBOOK™ SERIES
Giving Emergency Care Competently
Monitoring Fluid and Electrolytes Precisely
Assessing Vital Functions Accurately
Coping with Neurologic Problems Proficiently
Reading EKGs Correctly
Combatting Cardiovascular Diseases Skillfully

NURSE'S REFERENCE LIBRARY®
Diseases
Diagnostics
Drugs
Assessment
Procedures
Definitions
Practices

NURSING NOW™
Shock
Hypertension

NURSE'S CLINICAL LIBRARY™
Cardiovascular Disorders
Respiratory Disorders

Nursing84 **DRUG HANDBOOK™**

NURSING PHOTOBOOK™ Series

PUBLISHER
Eugene W. Jackson

EDITORIAL DIRECTOR
Jean Robinson

CLINICAL DIRECTOR
Barbara McVan, RN

ART DIRECTOR
Lisa A. Gilde

**Springhouse Corporation
Book Division**

DIRECTOR
Timothy B. King

DIRECTOR, RESEARCH
Elizabeth O'Brien

VICE-PRESIDENT, PRODUCTION AND PURCHASING
Bacil Guiley

Staff for this volume

BOOK EDITOR
Katherine W. Carey

SENIOR CLINICAL EDITOR
Paulette J. Strauch, RN

CLINICAL EDITORS
Mary L. Clements, RN, CCRN
Carol H. Best, RN, CNRN

ASSOCIATE EDITORS
Patricia K. Lawson
Dario F. Bernardini

SPECIAL ASSIGNMENTS EDITOR
Patricia R. Urosevich

PHOTOGRAPHER
Paul A. Cohen

ASSOCIATE DESIGNERS
Linda Jovinelly Franklin
Scott M. Stephens
Carol Stickles

ASSISTANT PHOTOGRAPHER
Thomas Staudenmayer

EDITORIAL/GRAPHIC COORDINATOR
Doreen K. Stowers

CLINICAL/GRAPHIC COORDINATOR
Evelyn M. James

COPY EDITOR
Sharyl D. Wolf

EDITORIAL STAFF ASSISTANT
Cynthia A. O'Connell

PHOTOGRAPHY ASSISTANT
Frank Margeson

ART PRODUCTION MANAGER
Robert Perry

ARTISTS
Virginia Crawford
Robert H. Renn
Sandra Simms
Louise Stamper
Joan Walsh
Robert Walsh
Ron Yablon

RESEARCHER
Vonda Heller

TYPOGRAPHY MANAGER
David C. Kosten

TYPOGRAPHY ASSISTANTS
Janice Auch Haber
Ethel Halle
Diane Paluba
Nancy Wirs

PRODUCTION MANAGERS
Wilbur D. Davidson
Robert L. Dean, Jr.

PRODUCTION ASSISTANT
Donald G. Knauss

ILLUSTRATORS
John Dougherty
Jean Gardner
Tom Herbert
Robert Jackson
Earl Parker
Dennis Schofield
Bud Yingling

SERIES GRAPHIC DESIGNER
John C. Isely

COVER PHOTO
Photographic Illustrations

**Clinical consultants
for this volume**

Candace Stiklorius, RN, BSN
Staff Development Instructor
Hospital of the University of Pennsylvania
Philadelphia

Roseanne K. Thompson, RN, BSN
Instructor
Division of Clinical Education
Anne Arundel General Hospital
Annapolis, Md.

Amended reprint, 1984
© 1982 by Springhouse Corporation,
1111 Bethlehem Pike, Springhouse, PA 19477
All rights reserved. Reproduction in whole or in part by any means whatsoever without permission of the publisher is prohibited by law.
Printed in the United States of America.

PB-041283

Library of Congress Cataloging in Publication Data

Main entry under title:

Caring for surgical patients.

(Nursing Photobook)
"Nursing82 books."
Bibliography: p.
Includes index.
1. Surgical Nursing—Handbooks, manuals, etc.
I. Springhouse Corporation II. Series. [DNLM:
1. Surgical nursing—Methods.   WY 161 C277]
RD99.24.C37   610.73'677   81-20269
ISBN 0-916730-43-3   AACR2

Contents

Introduction

Preparing the patient

Managing postoperative care

Performing special procedures

Dealing with complications

Contributors

At the time of original publication, these contributors held the following positions.

Susan M. Beidler is a medical/surgical instructor at Albright College in Reading, Pennsylvania. She is a BS degree graduate of Albright College and holds an MSN degree from Philadelphia's University of Pennsylvania. Ms. Beidler holds memberships in the American Association of Critical-Care Nurses, the American Nurses' Association, the Pennsylvania Nurses' Association, and Sigma Theta Tau.

Nancy Kennedy is assistant director of nursing/staff development at General Hospital of Virginia Beach, Virginia. Ms. Kennedy holds a BSN degree from Duke University, Durham, North Carolina, and an MSN degree from the University of Rhode Island, Kingston, Rhode Island.

Kristine M. Kroner is head nurse of the Urology Department at Albert Einstein Medical Center, Northern Division, in Philadelphia. A BSN degree graduate of Viterbo College in La Crosse, Wisconsin, Ms. Kroner is studying for an MS degree in health administration at Philadelphia's St. Joseph's University.

Suzanne D. Skinner is a lecturer at the University of Maryland School of Nursing in Baltimore. She holds BSN and MS degrees from the University of Maryland Baltimore Professional Schools. In addition, she earned a nursing diploma at the University of Virginia, Charlottesville, Virginia, and is a member of Sigma Theta Tau.

Candace Stiklorius is a staff development instructor at the Hospital of the University of Pennsylvania in Philadelphia, and an advisor for this PHOTOBOOK. A diploma graduate of the Hospital of the University of Pennsylvania School of Nursing in Philadelphia, she also holds a BSN degree from the University of Pennsylvania. Ms. Stiklorius is an MSN degree student at the University of Pennsylvania. In addition, she is a member of the American Nurses' Association, and the Pennsylvania Nurses' Association.

Roseanne K. Thompson, an advisor for this PHOTOBOOK, is an instructor in the Division of Clinical Education at Anne Arundel General Hospital in Annapolis, Maryland. She holds a BSN degree from the University of Maryland University City, College Park, Maryland.

Introduction

Never before has surgery been as safe and effective for patients as it is today. But, as a nurse, you know that refined surgical techniques and sophisticated medications provide no guarantees of success. Surgery, after all, is an invasive procedure. By its very nature, it poses risks for your patient. Clearly, your expert nursing care is as important now as it's ever been.

That's where this PHOTOBOOK comes in. Filled with the latest advice and techniques from our expert contributors, it provides just what you need to sharpen your skills.

As you know, surgical care begins long before your patient enters the operating room. That's why we've devoted the large first section to preparing your patient.

What does preparation mean? It should include preoperative assessment, history taking, testing, patient teaching, and routine procedures such as skin preparation. In the first section, you'll find essential information on all these topics, and more. And, in the appendices of this book, you'll find guidelines for interpreting routine preoperative test results.

Now, how about after surgery? If you work in the recovery room, you need to know how to monitor your patient's recovery from the anesthetic, and how to alleviate his pain. If you work in a medical/surgical nursing unit, you must know how to manage his ongoing recovery. Your responsibilities range from such seemingly-simple tasks as making a postoperative bed and giving a bed bath (are you *sure* you know the best techniques for these procedures?), to pain management and ambulation. We'll cover these subjects and many others in detail.

Of course, caring for your patient's surgical wound is one of your biggest challenges. Do you know how to change a dressing, using strict aseptic technique? How to apply a wet-to-dry dressing? And what if your patient has a draining wound—can you confidently evaluate the amount and color of drainage? Properly secure a dressing around a wound drain? Choose an appropriate drainage bag? Apply a skin barrier suitable for your patient's particular surgical wound? In the third section, you'll find all that you need to know.

Suppose, despite your best nursing care, your patient suffers a postoperative complication; for example, a wound infection, atelectasis, or shock. Can you recognize the problem, and adapt your nursing care to combat it? In the last section, we'll discuss the most common surgical complications, and show you how to cope with them.

No one has to tell you how important your job is. You know your patient depends on you for complete care, both before and after surgery. Use this PHOTOBOOK to assure yourself that you're giving him the very best care you can offer.

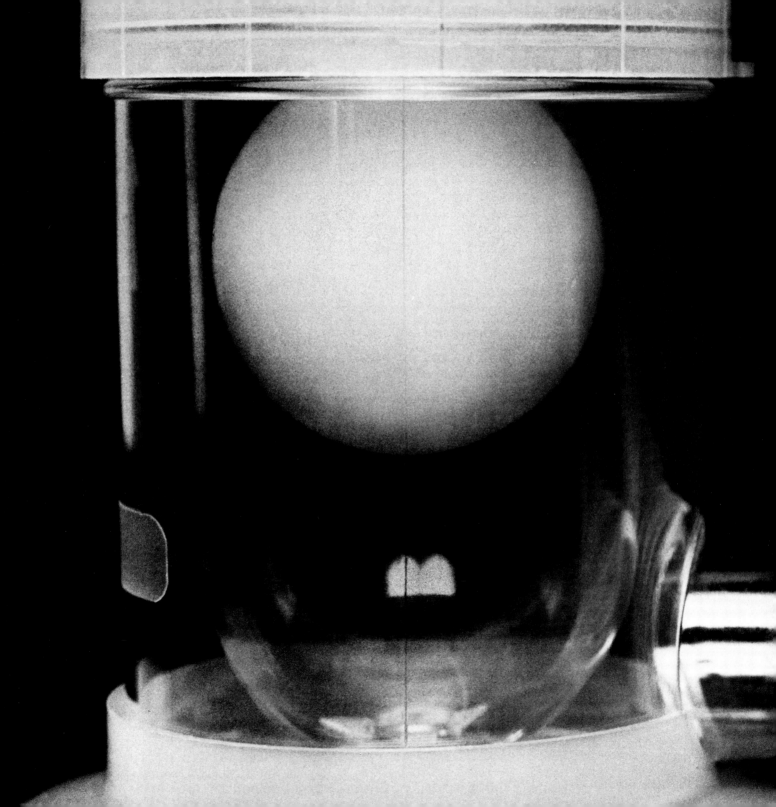

Preparing the Patient

Assessment

Testing

Patient teaching

Procedures

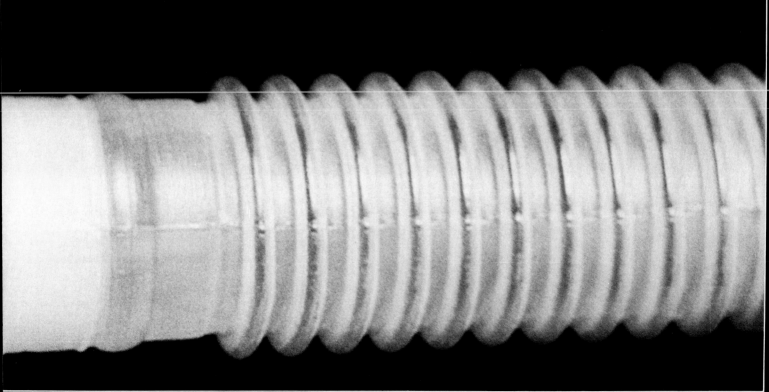

Assessment

Surgical care begins long before your patient enters the operating room. Consider a thorough preoperative assessment—one of your first nursing responsibilities when a surgical patient enters your care—to be the foundation of surgical care.

As you know, preoperative assessment provides a baseline for comparison throughout nursing care and medical treatment. But it can also help you identify conditions that impair the patient's ability to tolerate the stress of surgery, or to comply with postoperative routines. For example, if you discover that your patient's poorly nourished, you'll take special precautions to prevent pressure sores.

Throughout the assessment procedure, you'll stay alert for signs of psychological or social barriers to rapid recovery—depression, for example, or lack of emotional support from family or friends. And, of course, you'll update your initial assessment periodically as treatment progresses. Using this data base as a guide, you can tailor your nursing care to your patient's specific needs.

The surgical patient: A stranger in a strange land

"I've never been sick a day in my life," Todd Alvey tells you proudly. A self-employed carpenter, Mr. Alvey prides himself on his independence. A lifetime of hard work has enabled him to put three children through college, and provide a secure retirement for him and his wife. Now, at age 68, he finds himself admitted to the hospital for the first time, scheduled for a prostatectomy.

You can't help liking and admiring a patient like Mr. Alvey; he's so pleasant and undemanding. With his positive attitude, you may be tempted to conclude that he'll need no special emotional support while he's hospitalized. But think again. Behind his cheerful facade, he may be thinking: "Help me! I know nothing!"

Consider Mr. Alvey's feelings. He's never been hospitalized before, so all hospital routines and procedures are new and potentially frightening. In the next day or two, he'll be stuck with needles, poked and prodded, and bombarded with unfamiliar words and phrases. He'll be told what to eat, what not to eat, and when to eat. Even his urine will be scrutinized. In short, his independence will be compromised and his privacy invaded. Despite his calm outward appearance, he probably feels anxious, alone, and out-of-place—like a stranger in a strange land.

Preconceived notions

Mr. Alvey's feelings aren't surprising, especially if his impressions have been formed only by television programs and movies, or by limited personal experience. Soap operas, for example, show doctors and nurses dealing with personal problems, rather than performing patient care. Movies like *Coma* exploit commonly felt, if often unexpressed, fears of violation and powerlessness.

And what about his personal experiences with hospitals? Perhaps he visited one when his children were born, and another when his parents died. For him, the hospital is a place where life begins—and where it ends. Secretly, he may suspect he'll never awaken from the anesthetic.

Mr. Alvey has other concerns, too. For example, he faces a change in his body image. After all, he knows that surgery is an invasive procedure, one that'll leave a scar. For most patients, this thought alone is terrifying. Mr. Alvey also faces significant changes in his lifestyle and self-image. If the surgery leaves him sexually impotent, his relationship with his wife, and his own self-image, will be profoundly affected.

Although Mr. Alvey's only an example, his fears and concerns are common to most surgical patients—even those who've had surgery before. As a nurse, one of your most important responsibilities is to reduce your patients' emotional stress as much as possible. What can you do?

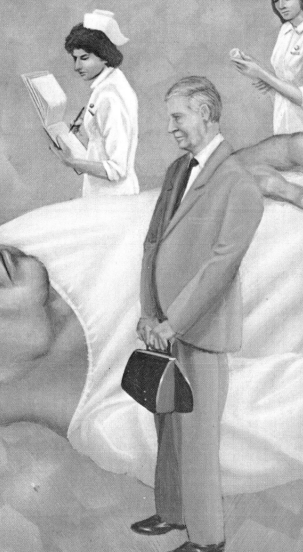

How you can help

Providing emotional support for a patient like Mr. Alvey may be difficult. Most likely, a man this age is reluctant to confess his fears and ask for help—especially if you're a female nurse who's young enough to be his daughter. But you can anticipate and relieve many of his fears with patient teaching. When your patient knows what to expect—before, during, and after surgery—he'll experience less fear of the unknown.

You can also correct any misconceptions your patient has. Mr. Alvey's concerns, for example, may be complicated by a basic ignorance of anatomy and physiology. No doubt, his doctor's explained that his prostate gland must be removed, and that the

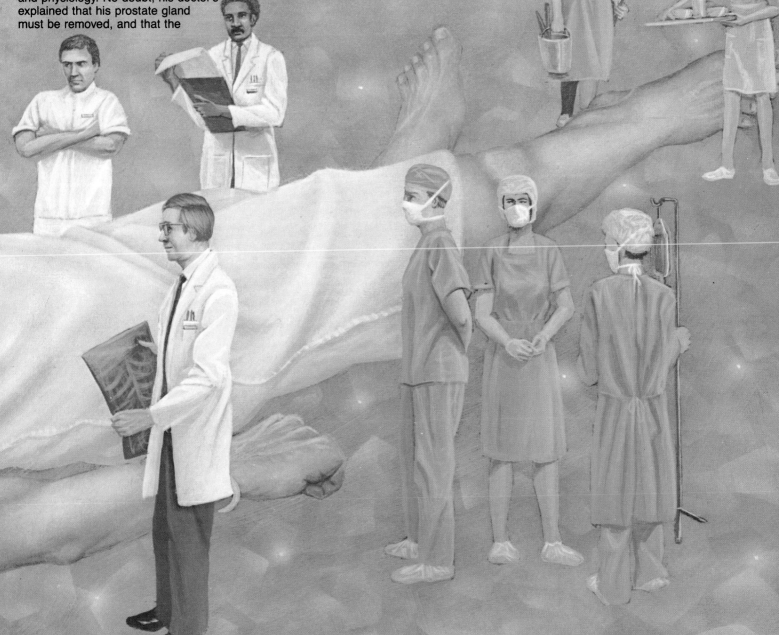

surgery may leave him sexually impotent. But Mr. Alvey may have no idea what his prostate gland is, where it's located—or how its removal will affect his appearance. You can help him understand.

Remember to talk to him in simple, easily-understood language. This means avoiding hospital jargon, as well as technical terms. For example, suppose you tell your patient something like this: "After you leave the recovery room, you'll be put back on the floor." *You* know exactly what you mean. But your patient may anticipate waking up on the floor—literally.

Assessment

The surgical patient: A stranger in a strange land continued

Accepting your limitations

Of course, many of your patient's fears are realistic, and can't be explained away. Recognize your limitations: You can't prevent or solve all the problems surgery may create in the short time your patient's in your care. But you can encourage your patient to express his concerns and ask you questions.

Never be afraid to admit that you don't know the answer to a question. Instead, tell your patient you'll find out for him.

Then, follow up.

Think back to Mr. Alvey. What if he feels too embarrassed to discuss sexual problems with you? Make sure he knows that sexual counseling is available, and explain how to get it. Or, consider giving him a patient-teaching pamphlet or printed handout that can answer his questions and direct him to appropriate counseling—when he's ready for it. Also, try approaching his wife and offering to answer her questions.

Patient teaching's an ongoing responsibility. Throughout this book, we'll share methods and techniques for teaching your surgical patients and their families.

If your patient's hospitalized for only a short time, he may absorb only a small portion of the information you give him. But if you spend time with him, recognize his concerns, and answer his questions, one message will surely get through—that you and the other health care professionals he depends on care about him. And that may be the most important thing he needs to know.

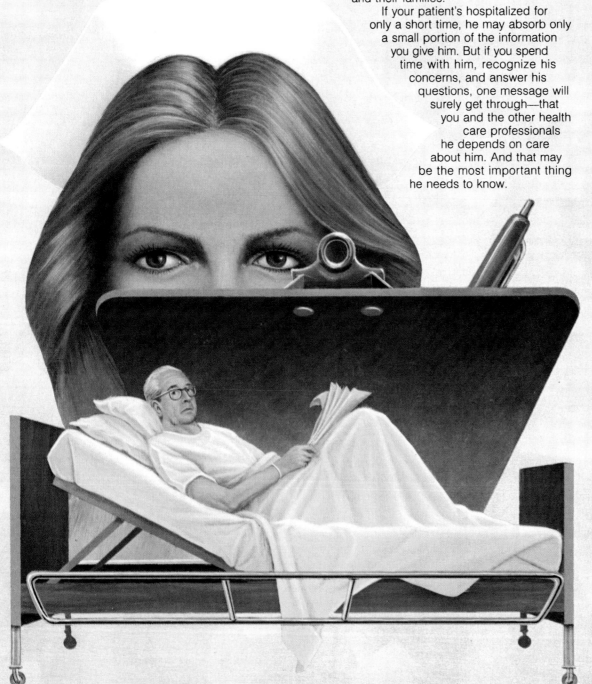

Tips for effective patient interviewing

How's your interviewing technique? Before you conduct your next interview, review these special tips. They'll help make each interview as productive as possible. *Note:* You can also use most of these techniques when conducting a physical examination or a patient-teaching session.

• Choose a time when neither you nor the patient is rushed, upset, or distracted.

• Provide a quiet, private setting. With the patient's permission, turn off the television or radio. Close his door or pull his curtain. But allow a family member to be present, if the patient wishes.

• Introduce yourself, and sit near the patient at his eye level. By sitting, you tell the patient that you're not in a hurry, and that you're interested in listening to him.

☎ *Nursing tip:* Avoid sitting in front of a window or bright light, or the patient will have to squint when he looks at you.

• Make sure that the patient's as comfortable as possible. For example, would he like another pillow? Does he need to go to the bathroom?

• Try to establish rapport with your patient. Stress the importance of the interview, and ask for his cooperation. Then, give him a chance to express his fears or ask questions *before* you begin the interview. After having this opportunity, he'll probably be more attentive to your questions.

- Avoid using medical terms or jargon. Stick to simple, readily-understood words and phrases. For example, don't say, "The doctor's ordered medication, p.r.n." Instead, say, "The doctor's ordered medication for you when you need and ask for it."
- Unless your patient is weak or short of breath, try to ask open-ended questions. For example, don't say, "Is the pain in your left side?" Instead, say, "Would you describe the pain's location for me?"
- Be a good listener. Don't interrupt the patient's answers. Encourage him to elaborate on them, when appropriate. When practical, document his own words.
- Keep the interview informal. However, don't let the patient wander too far off the track. If he begins to digress, tactfully lead him back to the subject with a comment like this: "Please tell me a little bit more about the headaches you've been having."
- Throughout the interview, remain receptive to the patient's questions and concerns. For example, he may wonder why you need to know about his bowel habits when he's hospitalized for cataract surgery. After you explain the importance of this information, he may be more cooperative.
- Remain nonjudgmental, no matter what the patient tells you. Your open, accepting attitude encourages the patient to be frank.

Interviewing your patient

When you're caring for a patient who's scheduled for surgery, take a complete, up-to-date health history as soon as possible. Try to conduct the interview before the physical examination, so you can examine problem areas with particular care. But keep in mind that the interview and the physical examination are closely related. Whenever appropriate, continue to question your patient about his condition as you conduct the physical examination. Thoroughly document your findings and observations, as well as the patient's own statements, on the form that your hospital provides.

Important: If your patient's unconscious, confused, or distracted by pain, ask his family or a friend for the information you need.

What do you need to learn from the patient interview? Use these topics as a guide:

Identity and chief complaint: Begin by asking the patient his name, address, age, and marital status. Then, record the patient's chief complaint. Using his own statement, your observations, and the admitting diagnosis, you'll be able to assess how well he understands his condition and the proposed surgical treatment.

Medical history: Ask the patient to describe any past illness, past surgery, injury, or other conditions; the approximate date of treatment; and his doctor's name. If he had surgery, did he experience any complications, such as pneumonia, shock, or wound infection?

Document any conditions that may affect your patient's tolerance to surgery, or his recovery. For example, is he diabetic? Does he have a bleeding disorder, heart disease, a seizure disorder, or a chronic respiratory condition?

Finally, document the patient's history of common childhood diseases, such as measles, mumps, and chicken pox.

Medications and allergies: Is your patient currently taking any medication? If so, document the medication's name and dosage, and the reason for its use. Because many medications interact with anesthetics or affect the patient's recovery, complete and accurate documentation is critical.

Note: Suppose your patient doesn't know the name of his medication. Ask him if he brought it with him. Maybe the hospital pharmacist or his family doctor can identify it. Or, if he didn't bring it, ask him to describe it for you, and find out why he uses it, and how often he takes it.

Next, find out if the patient's allergic to any medication, food, soaps, adhesive tape, iodine, insect stings, or pollen. Ask him to describe the type and severity of past allergic reactions. In addition, ask him to describe any adverse effects (such as dizziness, nausea, or diarrhea) that he's had from medications or food. (Keep in mind that a seafood allergy suggests sensitivity to iodine.)

Important: Note allergies in red on the appropriate form and the Kardex; also, flag the patient's chart. Then, place an allergy identification band on the patient's wrist.

Family health history: **Are the** patient's parents, siblings, or children alive? If so, are they in good health? If not, how old were they when they died, and what was the cause of death? Has anyone in his family ever had cancer, tuberculosis, diabetes, heart disease, chronic respiratory disease, kidney disease, or asthma?

Other considerations:
- his occupation and family structure. Is the patient employed outside the home? Note his occupation. Then, ask him to describe his family structure. Is he married? Do his children live with him? If he lives alone and has no family in the area, find out if a friend can help him after hospital discharge.
- his general health habits. Ask your patient to describe his eating habits. Does he follow any special diet? Note whether he's recently experienced any excessive weight loss or gain, and whether his current condition has affected his eating habits. In addition, ask him about his drinking, smoking, sleeping, and exercise patterns.
- any physical, mental, or language disabilities. Document anything that may limit the patient's ability to perform postoperative routines or to understand your patient teaching; for example, a hearing or sight impairment.
- prostheses or other artificial devices the patient uses. For example, document his use of glasses or contact lenses, artificial eyes or limbs, hearing aid, leg brace, dentures, ostomy appliance, wheelchair or cane, wig, or voice box. Take special note if any prosthetic device is essential for the patient's comfort.
- previous hospital experiences. Previous hospitalizations will affect your patient's attitudes and expectations. So, if your patient's been hospitalized before, ask him how he feels about the experience. By noting his attitudes now, you can better plan his nursing care.
- his emotional and psychological health. Determine if the patient is under any additional stress; for example, from a job loss or a recent death in the family. Then, note your observations of the patient's manner during the interview. Was he alert, well-oriented and cooperative? Did he seem depressed or highly anxious? Document your impressions as objectively as possible.

Finally, give the patient a chance to volunteer any other information that will help you make him comfortable.

Note: Keep in mind that some anxiety is normal for a patient who's anticipating surgery. So, if your patient seems inappropriately relaxed or unconcerned, consider the possibility that he's suppressing his fears. Such a patient may cope poorly with surgical stress.

Assessment

Conducting a head-to-toe physical exam

Have you documented your patient's history? If so, you're ready to conduct a preoperative physical examination.

You'll focus on problem areas suggested by the patient's history, and on any body system that'll be directly affected by the surgical procedure. (For more details on performing a complete physical assessment, see the NURSING PHOTOBOOK ASSESSING YOUR PATIENTS.)

Begin the examination by noting your patient's general appearance. Does he look healthy and well-nourished, or does he appear ill? Is he over- or underweight?

Next, record the patient's height, weight, and vital signs measurements. For accuracy, take blood pressure readings in both arms, and document the patient's position during the procedure. Update vital signs measurements at least twice a day throughout the preoperative period. These measurements will help you establish a baseline for your patient. (For information on interpreting vital signs measurements, see the chart on page 16.)

Now you're ready to systematically examine your patient, head-to-toe. Use the following chart as a guide.

Note: Don't rely on your observations alone. Remember to ask your patient appropriate questions throughout the physical examination.

Head and neck
• Check the patient's scalp for lesions or parasitic infection.
• Check his jugular veins for distention.
• Note the color of his sclerae. A yellowish color suggests jaundice.
• Evert his lower eyelid, and note the color of his conjunctivae. If this tissue looks pale, suspect anemia.
• Check his nose and throat for signs of upper respiratory infection.
• Assess his mouth for sores, ulcerations, or bleeding of tongue, gums, and cheeks. Check his lips for a bluish or gray color, which may suggest cyanosis.
• Check his neck for stiffness or cervical node enlargement.

Neurologic system
• Assess the patient's level of consciousness and orientation.
• Note whether his pupils are uniform in size and shape.
• Assess the patient's gross motor movements (for example, while standing or walking), and his fine motor movements (for example, while writing).
Important: If you know or suspect that your patient has a neurologic problem, conduct a complete neurologic exam, as shown in the NURSING PHOTOBOOK COPING WITH NEUROLOGIC DISORDERS.

Extremities and skin
• Look for changes in his skin color or temperature, suggesting impaired circulation. Check for cyanotic nailbeds and finger clubbing.
• Note skin lesions.
• Assess skin turgor for signs of dehydration.
• Check extremities for edema. Ask the patient if his feet, ankles, or fingers ever swell.
• Note hair distribution on the patient's extremities. Uneven hair distribution suggests poor peripheral circulation.
• Carefully palpate leg veins for varicosity.
• Check all peripheral pulses (radial, pedal, femoral, and popliteal). Remember to check them bilaterally.

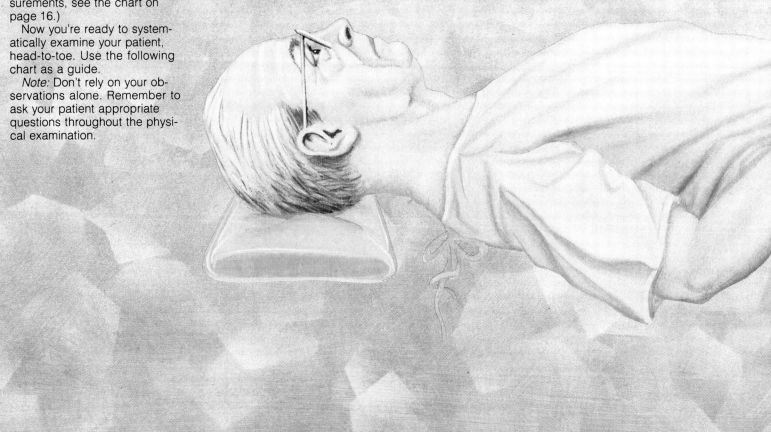

Respiratory system
- Document the patient's respiratory rate.
- Assess his breathing pattern. Inspect his chest wall for symmetry; look for use of accessory muscles.
- Auscultate his anterior and posterior chest for breath sounds. Listen for wheezing, coughing, and rales. Note dyspnea.

Cardiovascular system
- Assess his apical pulse for rate and regularity.
- Auscultate his heart sounds.
- Palpate his chest to find the point of maximal impulse (PMI).

Abdomen and gastrointestinal system
- Note the contour and symmetry of his abdomen; check for distention.
- Note position and color of his umbilicus; look for herniation.
- Auscultate his bowel sounds. Ask the patient if his bowel movements are regular.
- Percuss his abdomen for air and fluid.
- Palpate his abdomen for softness, firmness, and bladder height. Note any tenderness.
- Assess the six Fs: fat, fluid, flatus, feces, fetus (possibility of pregnancy), and fibroid tissue (or any unusual mass).

Genitourinary system
- Obtain a urine sample, if ordered; note its color and clearness.
- Ask the patient if he ever experiences pain, burning, or bleeding during urination. Does he frequently feel the need to urinate? Is he ever incontinent? Is he able to empty his bladder completely? Does he awaken at night to urinate?
- Note the general appearance of your patient's genitalia.
- If your patient's female, ask when her last menstrual period occurred, and find out if her cycle is regular. In addition, ask if she could possibly be pregnant.

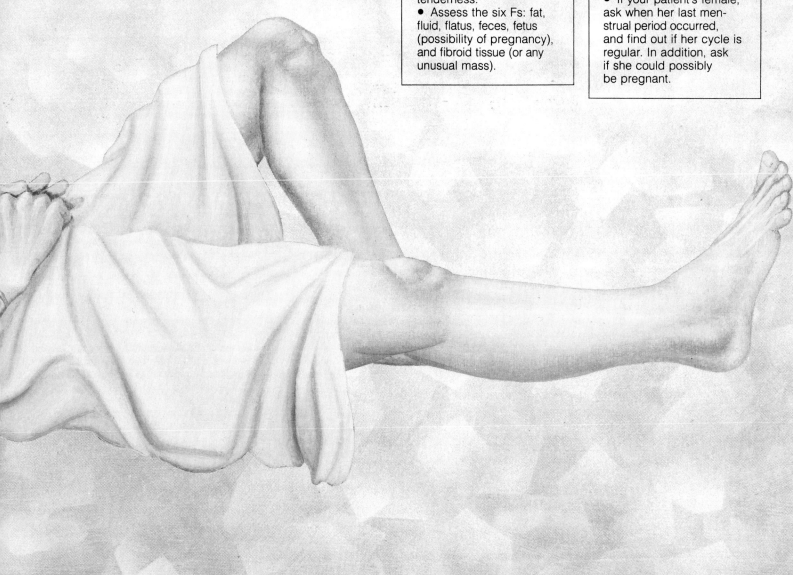

Assessment

Assessing your patient's vital signs

Vital signs measurements may suggest that your patient's at risk of postoperative complications. This chart tells you what vital signs variations may mean, and how they can affect your patient's tolerance to surgery. If your patient's vital signs are outside his normal limits, notify the doctor. He may treat the underlying cause, or postpone surgery until the patient's condition is stable.

Important: Use the measurements in this chart as guidelines only. Always consider what's normal for each patient. For example, low pulse rate and blood pressure may be normal in an athlete.

Vital sign	Abnormal finding	Possible indication	Possible postop complication
Temperature	Fever (above 101°F. [38.3°C.] in an adult)	Infection; dehydration (when accompanied by decreased skin turgor)	Systemic infection; wound infection, dehiscence, or evisceration; fluid imbalance; shock
Pulse	Tachycardia (above 100 beats per minute)	Pain; fever; dehydration; anemia; hypoxia; shock	Poor tissue perfusion; vascular collapse; cardiac arrhythmias; renal failure; anesthetic complications
	Bradycardia (below 60 beats per minute)	Drug effects (for example, of digitalis); spinal injury; head injury	Spinal shock; increased intracranial pressure. (See also complications for tachycardia listed directly above.)
Respiration	Tachypnea (above 24 breaths per minute)	Atelectasis; pneumonia; pain or anxiety; pleurisy; infection; renal failure	Tissue hypoxia; anesthetic complications; pneumonia; atelectasis
	Bradypnea (below 10 breaths per minute)	Brain lesion; respiratory center depression	See complications for tachypnea listed directly above.
Blood pressure	Hypotension (below 90 mm Hg systolic)	Shock; myocardial infarction; hemorrhage; spinal injury	Poor tissue perfusion; renal failure; vasodilation; shock
	Hypertension (above 140 mm Hg systolic and/or 90 mm Hg diastolic)	Anxiety or pain; renal disease; coronary artery disease	Stroke; hemorrhage; myocardial infarction

If your patient takes medications

If your patient regularly uses either prescription or over-the-counter medications, the doctor may adjust the dosage pre- or postoperatively—or temporarily discontinue the medication altogether.

Document *all* medications your patient's taken in the 2-week preoperative period (including birth control pills). Read what follows to learn about the possible effects of some commonly-used medications. (For details on specific medications, see the Nursing Drug Handbook™ or the Nurse's Guide to Drugs™.)

Anticoagulants: These medications increase the risk of hemorrhage. As a result, the doctor will discontinue anticoagulant therapy 48 hours before surgery, in most cases. If the patient's receiving heparin sodium (Lipo-Hepin), the doctor may reverse its anticoagulant effect with an antidote (such as protamine sulfate).

Antiarrhythmics: These medications may have significant effects while the patient's anesthetized. For example, propranolol hydrochloride (Inderal*) may depress myocardial function (resulting in decreased cardiac output and pulse rate), and induce

bronchospasm. Quinidine gluconate (Quinaglute Dura-Tabs*), procainamide hydrochloride (Pronestyl*), and lidocaine hydrochloride (Xylocaine*) may impair cardiac conduction, cause peripheral vasodilation, and potentiate anesthetics that act as neuromuscular blockades; for example, curare derivatives.

Antibiotics: When taken within 2 weeks of surgery, aminoglycoside antibiotics may produce mild respiratory depression from depressed neuromuscular transmission. During surgery, these medications seem to potentiate anesthetics that act as neuromuscular blockades.

Anticonvulsants: Long-term use of phenobarbital (Eskabarb*) and phenytoin sodium (Dilantin*) alters the metabolism of anesthetics. To compensate, the anesthesiologist may need to adjust the dosage and/or prolong the administration of the anesthetic.

Corticosteroids: After long-term use of corticosteroids, the patient's own adrenal glands won't function adequately. So, since surgery increases the demand for corticosteroids, the doctor will temporarily increase

the dosage before surgery.

Insulin: The diabetic patient's need for insulin will decrease preoperatively because he's fasting; after surgery, it may increase because of administration of dextrose and water I.V. during surgery. The doctor will closely monitor the patient's blood serum and urine sugar levels, and adjust the insulin dosage as needed.

Glaucoma medications: Some of these medications; for example, demecarium bromide (Humorsol) and echothiophate iodide (Phospholine Iodide*) have cumulative systemic effects, which may cause respiratory or cardiovascular collapse during surgery. They should be discontinued 10 to 14 days before surgery.

Antihypertensives: These medications inhibit the synthesis and storage of norepinephrine in sympathetic nerve endings, altering the patient's response to muscle relaxants and narcotic analgesics. The result may be hypotensive crisis during surgery or in the immediate postop period. The doctor may reduce or discontinue the dosage prior to surgery.

*Available in both the United States and in Canada

Testing

If your patient enters the hospital a day or more before surgery, he'll probably undergo routine preoperative tests: blood tests, chest X-rays, an electrocardiogram (if indicated), and a urinalysis. And if the diagnosis is uncertain, the doctor may also order further diagnostic tests.

In the following pages, you'll learn:
• how to prepare your patient for the routine preoperative tests he'll undergo.
• how to perform nursing procedures related to these tests, such as obtaining blood and urine specimens.
• how to prepare your patient for some common diagnostic tests.

As a nurse, you must also be able to evaluate routine test results. For guidance, turn to this book's appendix.

Teaching your patient about X-rays

Let's say your patient, Mr. Rubin, is scheduled for posterior-anterior (PA) chest X-rays prior to abdominal surgery. Since he's not on bed rest, he'll go to the X-ray department for the procedure. Your responsibility is to explain the procedure before he goes.

Even if Mr. Rubin's had X-rays before, don't assume he really understands them. Assess his level of knowledge; then, supplement or correct his information as necessary. Follow these guidelines:
• Tell the patient why the doctor's ordered a chest X-ray. For example, say something like this: "The doctor's ordered a chest X-ray so he can better evaluate your lungs and heart before surgery." Remember, the patient may incorrectly assume that he needs an X-ray because of a problem with his heart or lungs.
• Explain the procedure. Tell him that the X-ray technician will take X-rays of his chest from the back. For best results, the technician will ask the patient to stand with his hands on his hips.
• Describe the equipment he'll see. Remember, he may become apprehensive when he sees the large, unfamiliar machinery.
• Assure him that he'll receive only a small amount of radiation, and that the procedure's entirely safe. Explain that others in the room will shield themselves from the radiation because they're exposed to many X-rays each day.
• Is your patient a woman? Ask her when she had her last menstrual period. If there's any chance she's pregnant, ask the X-ray technician to shield the patient's uterus. Then, advise the patient of this special precaution.
• Warn the patient that the X-ray plate will feel cold.
• Tell him that he'll hear thudding sounds as the X-ray plates are changed.
• Encourage questions, and answer them completely and frankly.
• Ask him to remove jewelry and any other metal objects he's wearing above his waist. Explain that the metal will block the X-rays.
• Then, remove his clothing from the waist up and dress him in a hospital gown (or an X-ray gown, according to hospital policy). Tie the gown in the back, not the front. *Note:* Don't use a gown with metal snaps, because the snaps will show up on the X-rays and may look like abnormalities.
• Tell your patient to stand erect during the procedure, and to inhale deeply and hold his breath at the technician's request.

Using a portable X-ray machine

What if your surgical patient can't go to the X-ray department for some reason? The doctor may order a preop chest X-ray taken with a portable machine, even though it can only X-ray the anterior-posterior (AP) view. Here's what you should do to help:
• Prepare the patient as you would for a standard X-ray in the X-ray department. Follow the guidelines listed above.
• Raise the head of the bed as high as possible, or as high as the patient can comfortably tolerate.
• Tell the patient that the X-ray plate will feel cold.
 Nursing tip: For the patient's comfort, cover the X-ray plate with a pillowcase.
• Help the X-ray technician center the X-ray plate under the

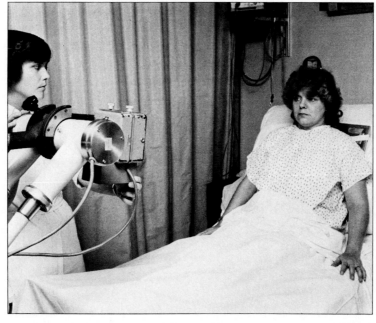

patient's back.
• Urge the patient to inhale deeply and hold her breath when the technician tells her to do so. *Important:* For safety, stand clear of the X-ray machine when X-rays are being taken—preferably behind a lead apron or out of the room. Make sure others do, too. This precaution's especially important for girls, and women of childbearing age.
• Document the procedure on the patient's chart and in your nurses' notes. Since the anterior-posterior (AP) view may distort the heart's size, be sure to note that the X-ray was taken with a portable X-ray machine. Clearly document the patient's position, too. A recumbent position changes the heart's position in the thorax.

Testing

Chest X-rays: What they reveal

No wonder preoperative chest X-rays are routine for most surgical patients. These valuable diagnostic tools can show the doctor the size and shape of the heart, lungs, aorta, and other large mediastinal structures; calcification in the heart and blood vessels; and fluid in the pleural spaces.

Take a look at the two examples below. The X-ray at left shows normal, disease-free heart and lungs. Now, contrast this with the X-ray at right. As you see, atelectasis has developed in the right middle lobe, causing it to completely collapse. (Note the central venous catheter in the superior vena cava.)

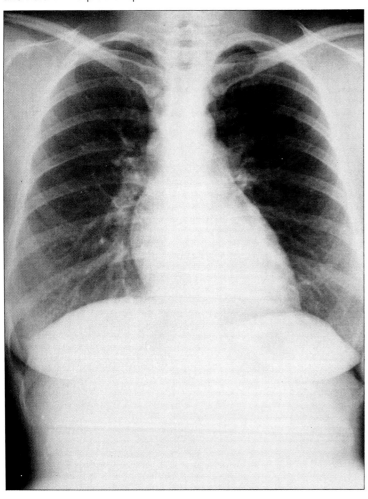

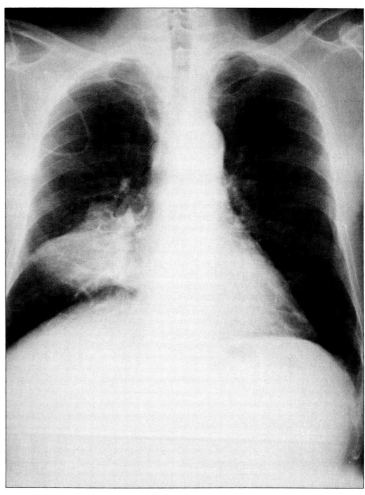

PATIENT PREPARATION

Collecting a urine specimen

Before your patient undergoes surgery, you'll request at least one urine specimen. In most cases, you'll teach the patient how to collect one himself.

To do so, give the patient a copy of one of the self-care aids on the following pages. Then, discuss the procedure with him, stressing the steps necessary to avoid contamination. Emphasize that he must obtain a mid-stream specimen.

Note: If possible, ask him to collect a first morning specimen. Because a first morning specimen is more concentrated than a later specimen, it's likely to yield more accurate test results. Also, its higher acidity helps preserve some urine components.

Suppose your female patient is menstruating. Ask her to gently place a cotton ball in her vaginal opening before obtaining the specimen. Note on the lab slip that the patient is menstruating.

Is your patient's urine production low? Unless contraindicated, suggest that he drink 1 or 2 cups of fluid at least 30 minutes before collecting the specimen.

Nursing tip: If the patient has difficulty urinating, suggest that he run water while preparing to collect the specimen.

Ask the patient to give you the specimen as soon as he's collected it. Then, label it and send it to the lab. For best results, the urine should be analyzed within 30 minutes after collection. However, if necessary, you may refrigerate it for up to 2 hours.

Self-care

How to collect a urine specimen (for the male patient)

1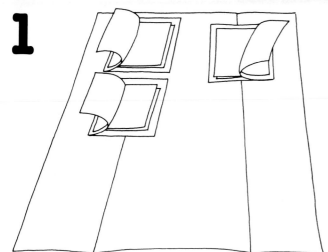

Dear Patient:
The doctor's ordered a routine test of your urine, to see how well your kidneys and urinary tract are working. To make sure the results are accurate, carefully follow these directions.

First, wash your hands. Open a paper towel on a nearby clean, dry surface. Then, open the three disposable wipes, and place them on the towel, as shown here.

2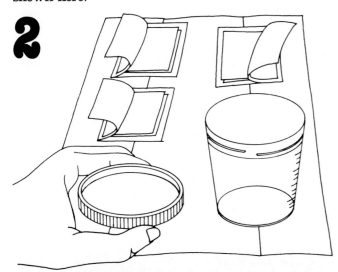

Without touching the insides of the plastic specimen cup or the lid, remove the lid from the cup. Place the cup on the paper towel. Lay the lid next to it, flat side down.

3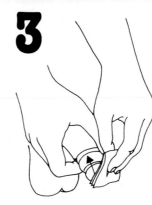

Grasp your penis, as if you were going to urinate. If you're uncircumcised, pull back your foreskin. Then, use the three disposable wipes to clean the head of your penis. Clean from the urethral opening toward you, as shown. Discard each wipe as soon as you've used it. Pick up the cup. (Remember not to touch its inside.)

4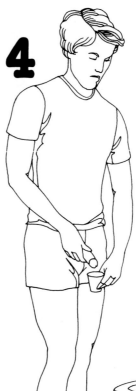

Urinate a small amount into the toilet or urinal; then, stop the flow. Hold the cup a few inches away from your penis, taking care not to touch the inside of the cup with your penis or fingers. Urinate into the cup, until it's about two-thirds full. Don't let the cup overflow. Place the cup on the paper towel, and finish urinating, if necessary. Then, replace the lid on the cup (without touching the lid's inside), and return the cup to the nurse.

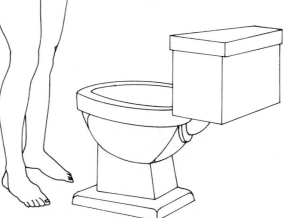

Testing

Self-care

How to collect a urine specimen (for the female patient)

1

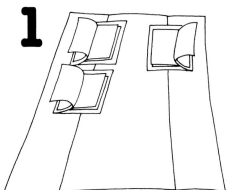

Dear Patient:
The doctor's ordered a routine test of your urine, to see how well your kidneys and urinary tract are working. To make sure the results are accurate, carefully follow these directions.

First, remove all your clothes from the waist down, and wash your hands thoroughly. Open a paper towel on a nearby clean, dry surface. Then open the three disposable wipes and place them on the towel, as shown here.

2

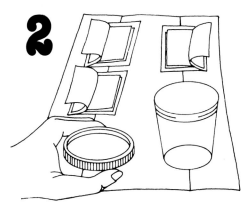

Without touching the inside of the plastic specimen cup or the lid, remove the lid from the cup. Place the cup on the paper towel. Lay the lid next to it, flat side down.

3

Sit as far back on the toilet as possible, and spread your legs apart. Then, using your fingertips, separate your labia (the skin around the urethral opening). This drawing shows where your labia and other nearby body parts are located. Keep the labia separated for the rest of the procedure.

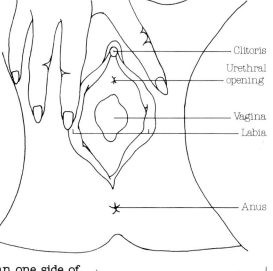

Clitoris
Urethral opening
Vagina
Labia
Anus

4

Use a wipe to clean one side of your labia, with a single top-to-bottom stroke, and discard the wipe. Take another wipe, and repeat the procedure on the other side of the labia. Then, use the third wipe to clean the urethral opening. Discard the wipe, and pick up the cup. (Remember not to touch its inside.)

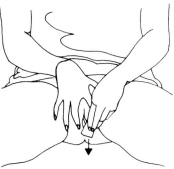

5

Urinate a small amount into the toilet. Then, stop the flow, and hold the cup as shown here. Urinate into the cup until it's about two-thirds full. Be careful not to let the cup overflow. Place the filled cup back on the paper towel and finish urinating, if necessary.

Securely place the lid on the cup, taking care not to touch the inside of the cup or lid with your fingers. Wash your hands, and get dressed. Return the filled cup to the nurse.

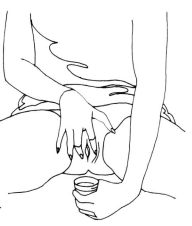

Aspirating a urine specimen

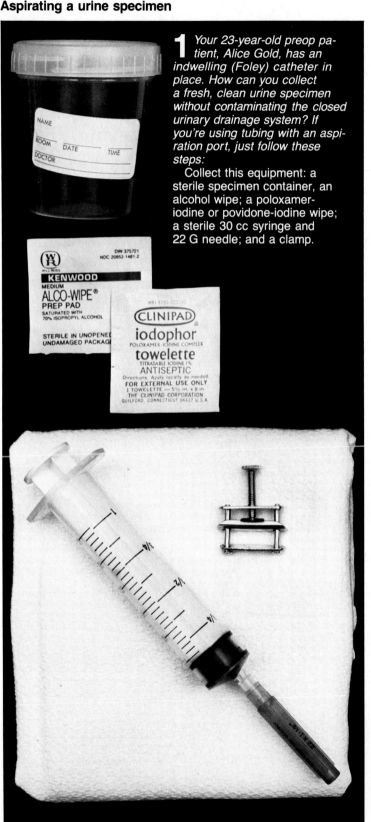

1 *Your 23-year-old preop patient, Alice Gold, has an indwelling (Foley) catheter in place. How can you collect a fresh, clean urine specimen without contaminating the closed urinary drainage system? If you're using tubing with an aspiration port, just follow these steps:*

Collect this equipment: a sterile specimen container, an alcohol wipe; a poloxamer-iodine or povidone-iodine wipe; a sterile 30 cc syringe and 22 G needle; and a clamp.

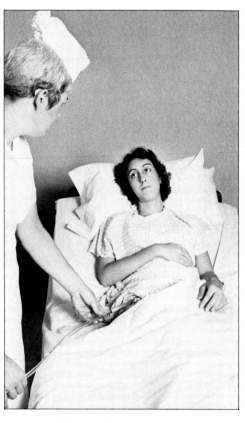

2 Tell the patient that you're collecting a routine preop urine sample. Then, to ensure a fresh urine sample, straighten the drainage tubing to drain all urine into the drainage bag.

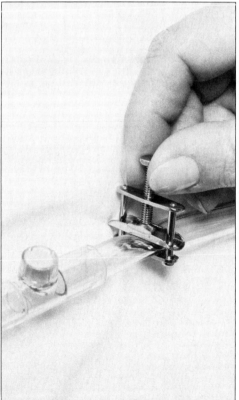

3 Now, clamp the drainage tubing below the aspiration port, as shown in the photo. In about 10 to 30 minutes, enough urine will accumulate for an adequate specimen (10 to 30 ml). Place a sign above the patient's bed stating the time you clamped the tubing. Check the drainage tubing every 10 minutes to assess urine production.

Testing

Aspirating a urine specimen continued

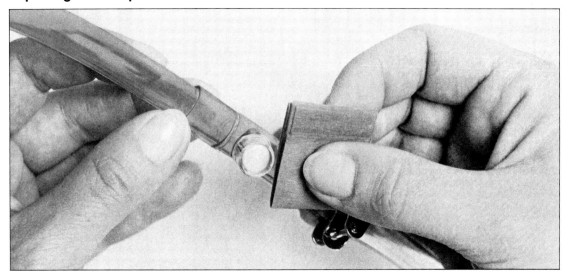

4 When enough urine has collected in the tubing, wash your hands. Then, using the povidone-iodine wipe, thoroughly clean the aspiration port with a brisk, rubbing motion that creates friction. Clean the port for 1 minute. Then, use the alcohol wipe to clean the povidone-iodine from the port.

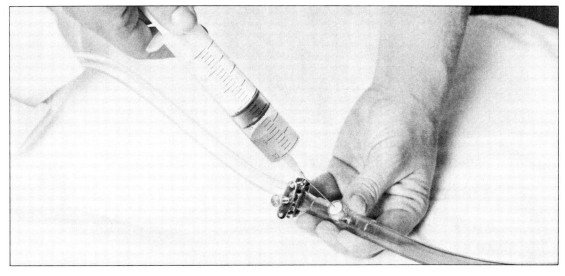

5 Next, expel the air in the syringe, and puncture the aspiration port with the needle. Aspirate about 30 ml of urine, if possible.

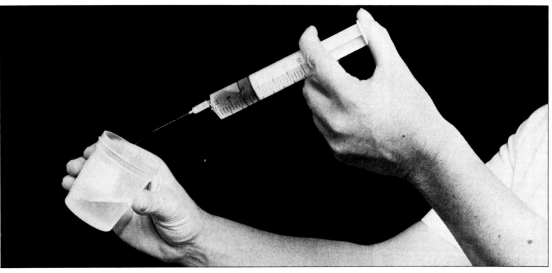

6 Withdraw the needle from the port and expel the urine into the clean specimen container. To avoid contaminating the specimen, don't allow the needle to touch the inside of the cup. Also, minimize the airspace the specimen passes through. Put the lid on the specimen container, and label the container. Send the specimen to the lab, and document the procedure. *Important:* Remember to unclamp the tubing, and discard the sign you placed above the patient's bed.

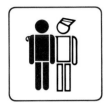

Preparing your patient for venipuncture

For you, obtaining a blood specimen may seem like one of the least complicated preoperative procedures that your patient experiences. But your patient may think otherwise, especially if he's frightened by the sight of needles or blood. So, always prepare your patient for venipuncture. Keep these points in mind:

• Tell him why blood specimens are needed.
• Explain to him that several blood specimens can be taken during a single venipuncture.
• Reassure him that the amount of blood taken is very small.
• Tell him that his body will quickly replace the blood you've taken.
• Give him tips for reducing discomfort during the procedure. For example, advise him to relax as much as possible, and to take a deep breath as the needle punctures his skin. Emphasize that the discomfort lasts only a short time.

If possible, perform venipuncture in a quiet setting, to help your patient relax. If he remains anxious, despite your efforts, consider postponing the procedure until he's calmer. Remember, anxiety causes the veins to constrict, making venipuncture more difficult. For some patients, the doctor may order a mild sedative.

In the photostory beginning on page 24, you'll see how to obtain blood specimens. For more details on performing venipuncture, see the NURSING PHOTO-BOOK MANAGING I.V. THERAPY.

Choosing a site for venipuncture

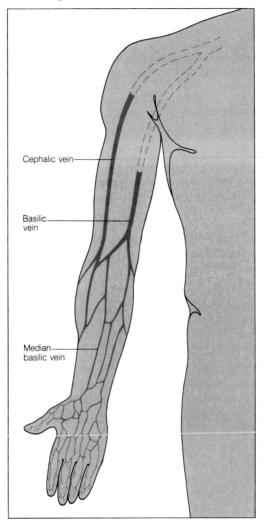

Cephalic vein

Basilic vein

Median basilic vein

What's the best site for obtaining blood specimens? For most adult patients, a vein in the antecubital fossa is best. (See the illustration at left.) But you may also consider a vein in another part of the arm, or in the hand. For the patient's comfort, use his nondominant hand or arm, if possible. (But, avoid using his legs, since they're prone to complications such as phlebothrombosis (clotting in a vein without inflammation of the vein wall).

Note: If you're withdrawing blood from a vein in the patient's hand, use a small-gauge needle and syringe, instead of the Vacutainer® collection tubes featured in the following photostory. Doing so reduces the risk of rupturing the vein during venipuncture.

Look for a vein that's full, soft, and unobstructed. Palpate to find one that's not crooked, hardened, scarred, or inflamed. If you must use the patient's leg, be sure to check it carefully for varicosity *above* the venipuncture site.

Before choosing a vein, consider these additional factors:

• Does the patient already have an I.V. in place? If so, choose a vein in the opposite extremity.
• Does your patient have a condition, such as hemiplegia, that affects one side of his body? Choose a vein on the opposite side. Circulation to his affected extremity is already impaired through disuse. *Note:* Suppose such a patient has an I.V. catheter inserted in his unaffected arm. Apply the tourniquet *below,* not above, the I.V. site. Then, obtain the blood specimens from a site *below* the tourniquet.

How to dilate a vein

Planning to perform venipuncture? Make this procedure as quick and comfortable as possible for the patient by using the following tips for dilating a vein:

• Position selected limb below heart level.
• Apply digital pressure just above the selected insertion site. If the patient's veins are large and prominent, this simple technique raises a vein quickly. Then, apply a tourniquet.
• If applying a tourniquet doesn't fully engorge the vein, ask the patient to open and close his fist repeatedly. Ask him to close his fist as you insert the needle and to open it again when the needle's in place.
• If your patient's too weak to energetically clench and unclench his fist, apply a second tourniquet over his wrist or hand.
• Or, place your fingers over the vein be-

tween the tourniquet and the venipuncture site, and use short, stroking motions to milk it down against the blood flow.
• If these methods don't work, try heat. Wrap the entire limb in warm, wet towels (or a heating pad) for 10 to 20 minutes before applying the tourniquet. Maintain the heat by wrapping the toweling in a bed-saver pad or plastic bag. (For maximum vein engorgement, lower the patient's limb over the bed's side for 2 or 3 minutes. But watch the patient carefully, and observe the distal end of the limb for discoloration.)

When the veins are engorged, apply a tourniquet and perform venipuncture. *Important:* Never tightly apply a tourniquet when the veins are engorged. This may cause the vein to rupture during venipuncture.

Testing

Drawing blood specimens in proper sequence

Collecting blood specimens? Avoid jeopardizing test results, by filling the collection tubes in proper sequence.

The laboratory will give you collection tubes to use. You can identify them by their color-coded stoppers. Check the lab manual for your hospital's color code. Then, follow these guidelines:
• Fill sterile blood culture tubes first, to minimize the risk of contaminating the specimen. These tubes contain a culture medium.

• Next, fill empty tubes (those that don't contain anticoagulant additives). This way, the blood can begin clotting while you work.
• Last, fill tubes that contain anticoagulant additives, such as oxalates or heparin. These additives appear as white powder or clear liquid. After filling these tubes, gently rotate them five or six times, to thoroughly mix the blood and additives.

Obtaining blood specimens

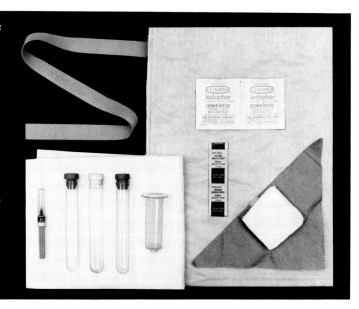

1 In most hospitals, lab technicians usually obtain the blood specimens from preoperative patients. But in an emergency, or when the hospital's short-staffed, you may have to do the procedure. Make sure you know how by reviewing the following steps. (Note: Some tests, such as coagulation studies, require special procedures. Expect a lab technician to perform such tests.)

If possible, plan to obtain blood specimens before the patient has breakfast, or at least 6 hours after a meal. If your patient has had a large meal within the last 4 to 12 hours, take care to document this on the lab slip.

What equipment do you need? First, find out what tests the doctor's ordered. Then, check your hospital lab manual to learn how many collection tubes you'll need, and what size they should be. In this photostory, we'll assume that you need the equipment shown here: three Vacutainer® collection tubes (two empty; one containing an anticoagulant), a Vacutainer® sterile needle and sleeve, poloxamer-iodine or povidone-iodine wipes, sterile 2″ x 2″ gauze sponges, tourniquet, bed-saver pad, and an adhesive bandage strip. (If necessary, also include a lamp to assure adequate lighting.) *Important:* Is your patient allergic to iodine? Use alcohol wipes instead.

2 Unless contraindicated, place the patient in a supine position with the head of the bed elevated and her lower arms and hands resting on the bed. This position encourages vein engorgement in the extremities. Place the bed-saver pad under the patient's arm, and explain the procedure to her. (Follow the guidelines on page 23.)

Thoroughly wash your hands. Screw the Vacutainer needle into the sleeve, as shown in the inset photo. Lay the needle and sleeve on a nearby clean surface.

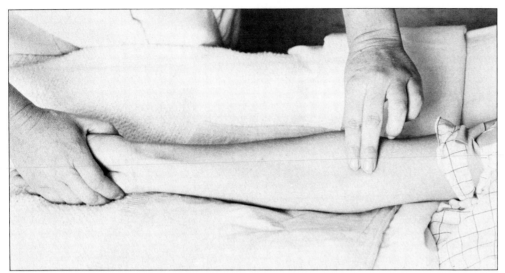

3 Apply a tourniquet to the patient's arm. Avoid pinching the patient's skin, by tucking a part of her gown sleeve under the tourniquet, as shown here. Then, palpate to select a suitable vein. (For guidance on vein selection, see the illustration on page 23.) If your patient's veins are small, ask her to clench and unclench her fist as you palpate. Or, obtain a small-gauge needle.

When you've selected a vein, release the tourniquet. By releasing the tourniquet, you avoid prolonged venous obstruction. Prolonged venous obstruction may generate high pressure in the vein, causing it to rupture during venipuncture. Prolonged venous pressure may also cause hemolysis, which can alter test results.

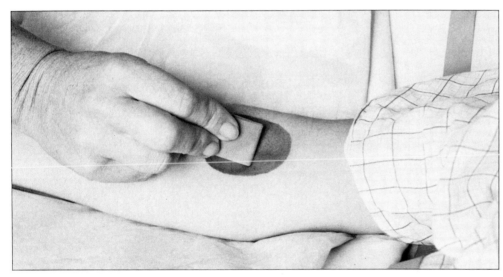

4 Using a brisk circular motion, clean the venipuncture site for 1 minute with the poloxamer-iodine wipe. (If you're cleaning the skin with alcohol instead of poloxamer-iodine, continue the cleansing procedure for 3 minutes.) Begin at the puncture site and work outward. Discard the wipe, and wait about 30 seconds for the skin to dry. (Don't wave your hand above the site to dry it, or you'll increase the risk of contamination.) *Important:* When you've completed the procedure, do not touch the site again.

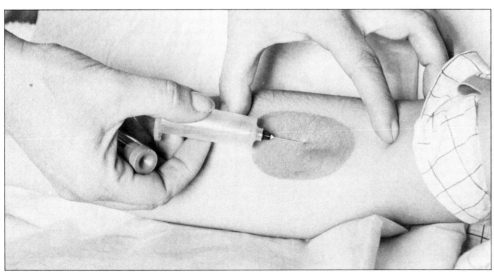

5 Now, reapply the tourniquet to her arm 2″ to 6″ above the venipuncture site. Tighten the tourniquet enough to impede venous flow without stopping arterial flow. Then, position her arm so it's level and firmly supported, as the nurse has done here. Ask the patient to remain still.

Remove the needle cover. Then, holding the needle so the lumen faces up, insert the needle into the patient. If you've entered the vein properly, you'll see a drop of blood at the end of the needle in the sleeve. If you haven't entered the vein properly, withdraw the needle and prepare to begin the procedure again, at another site. *Important:* If you fail to obtain blood after two tries, ask someone who's more experienced at venipuncture to take over.

Testing

Obtaining blood specimens continued

6 Now you're ready to begin filling the tubes. Take care to fill them in the proper order, as outlined at the top of page 24.

Gently push an empty collection tube into the needle sleeve, until the needle penetrates the tube's stopper. Blood will immediately begin filling the tube. Stabilize the vein with your nondominant hand, so the needle doesn't perforate the vein's opposite wall.

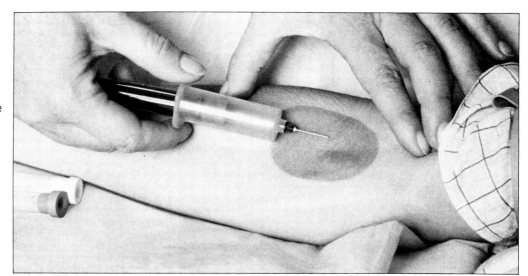

7 When the tube's full, use your free hand to remove the tube and replace it with the next empty one. (Some blood may drip from the needle's end as you do so.) Repeat the procedure to fill the tube containing the anticoagulant, as shown here. *Note:* Some Vacutainer tubes are designed to fill only partially. Remove these tubes as soon as blood ceases to flow into the tube.

Release the tourniquet when the third tube is about three-quarters full. Then, continue to fill the tube, and remove the needle, as explained below. By releasing the tourniquet a short time before removing the needle, you reduce the risk of hematoma formation at the venipuncture site after needle removal. In addition, you reduce the chance of hemolysis, which may alter test results.

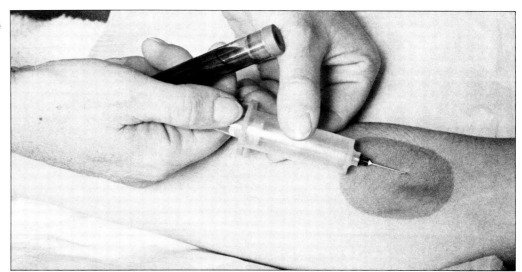

8 When you've released the tourniquet and finished filling the last tube, use this procedure to remove the needle: Lightly hold a clean gauze sponge over the vein, slightly above the tip of the needle. Withdraw the needle from the vein at the same angle you inserted it. As you do, slide the sponge down the vein, so that it covers the venipuncture site, and apply direct pressure.

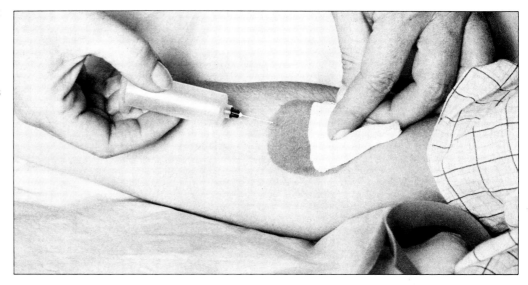

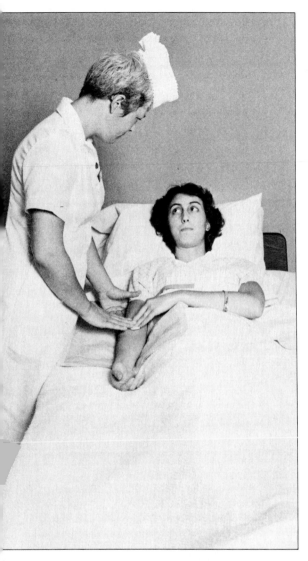

9 If possible, ask the patient to hold the sponge, applying direct pressure to the venipuncture site. Ask her to maintain this position for about 1 minute, or until bleeding stops. (Don't ask her to bend her elbow and hold her arm up, because this may increase the risk of bruising.)

Important: If your patient has an abnormal clotting time, or is taking anticoagulants, ask her to apply direct pressure for at least 3 minutes, or until bleeding stops.

Remain with the patient until bleeding stops. While you wait, gently invert the tube containing anticoagulant five or six times. (Do not vigorously shake the tube.) Then, label the tubes and fill out the necessary lab slips.

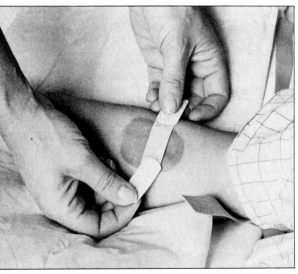

10 When bleeding stops, apply an adhesive bandage strip to the venipuncture site. Ask the patient to avoid strenuous use of this arm for a few hours to prevent bleeding. If your patient has an abnormal clotting time, frequently check the venipuncture site.

Send the specimens to the lab immediately. Document the procedure.

Preparing your patient for a 12-lead EKG

Will your patient undergo preoperative electrocardiography? That depends—on your patient's condition, the doctor's preference, and hospital policy. But if he *is* scheduled for a routine electrocardiogram (EKG), make sure you prepare him by carefully explaining the procedure beforehand.

Suppose your patient's never had an EKG before. He may suspect that the electrodes and wires will give him an electrical shock. Or, he may worry that he needs the procedure because he's having a heart attack.

Spare your patient needless anxiety. First, assure him that the test is completely painless. Explain that the procedure's routine for patients scheduled for surgery, and that it doesn't necessarily indicate a problem with his heart. Then, take time to explain the procedure to him. If he's had an EKG before, find out how much he understands about it; then, supplement his information.

Here are some questions your patient's likely to have, and some suggested answers. To help the patient understand your answers, consider giving him EKG waveform strips and electrodes to examine.

Patient's question: What *is* an EKG?

Your answer: The term EKG (or ECG) is an abbreviation for electrocardiogram. When interpreted by a trained person, the EKG shows your heart's electrical activity. Approximately once each second, a specialized group of heart cells, forming the sinus node, releases an electrical current that spreads throughout your heart. This current stimulates your heart to beat. Then, it spreads throughout your whole body, although you don't feel it. The EKG electrodes that will be applied to your skin pick up this current. Then, the EKG machine records the current as waveforms on a long strip of paper, called an EKG waveform strip. Here's what one looks like.

Patient's question: What are electrodes?

Your answer: For your EKG, I'll apply two different types. The electrodes I'll put on each of your arms and legs are small metal rectangles that look like this. They're held in place with rubber straps. I'll put a fifth electrode on your chest; it's held in place by suction, so it has a rubber bulb on top of it.

I'll put a special jelly under each electrode to help it pick up your heart's electrical signals clearly. This jelly may feel cold at first. I'll wipe it off after the test.

Patient's question: Why so many electrodes?

Your answer: The four electrodes on your arms and legs allow the EKG machine to record electrical current from six different directions. The chest electrode, which I'll reposition several times during the procedure, provides six additional views for a total of twelve views. These twelve views of the heart provide a nearly complete picture of the heart's electrical activity.

Patient's question: Can this equipment give me a shock?

Your answer: No. EKG equipment only measures electrical activity normally present in your body; it does not transmit any electricity into your body.

Patient's question: How long does the EKG take?

Your answer: After the electrodes are in place, the procedure takes less than 5 minutes.

Patient's question: What do I do during the procedure?

Your answer: Just lie flat and relax. Breathe normally and keep your arms and legs still. And don't talk—talking may distort the waveforms.

Testing

Common diagnostic X-rays

To confirm his preoperative diagnosis, the doctor may order one or more X-ray tests. The chart below describes some of those most commonly performed.

If your patient's scheduled for any diagnostic test, take the time to explain the procedure to him, and answer his questions. Make sure he understands the anatomical structures involved, as well as the test's purpose. Use simple, nontechnical terms, but be sure to explain any medical or nursing terms he's likely to hear; for example, NPO (nothing by mouth).

Keep in mind that procedures vary from hospital to hospital. Learn your hospital's specific requirements for each procedure, so you don't misinform or confuse your patient. *Note:* Notify both the doctor and the X-ray technician if your patient's pregnant. They may decide not to expose the fetus to X-rays, or they may provide a lead apron to protect the fetus. Also, tell your patient to remind the X-ray technician that she's pregnant.

Upper GI series

Purpose
To examine the esophagus, stomach, and small intestine, and to identify upper gastrointestinal (GI) tract disorders, such as tumors, ulcers, and swallowing malfunctions

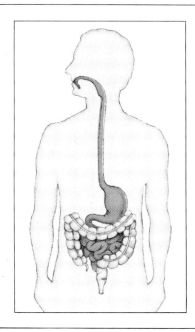

What to tell the patient
The doctor wants to take X-rays of your throat, stomach, and small intestine. You will go to the X-ray department, where the doctor or technician will ask you to drink a liquid called barium. It's a flavored liquid with a chalky consistency, similar to flavored Milk of Magnesia. The barium coats your digestive tract, which then shows up clearly on X-ray film. As the barium passes through your digestive tract, the doctor will take X-rays from many angles, at 15 to 30 minute intervals.

The doctor may also ask you to swallow some flavored granules. These granules produce air in your stomach and help it show up better on X-rays. Or, the doctor may ask you to drink a carbonated drink, which has the same effect. You may feel like burping, but try not to do so until the procedure is finished.

If the doctor wants to examine your entire small intestine, he'll ask you to drink several more cups of barium solution. The entire test will take between 1 and 4 hours. The doctor may ask you to wait in the X-ray department while he examines the film; if necessary, he'll take more X-rays before you return to your room.

Because food in your digestive tract would make the X-rays hard to interpret, you'll have only a clear-liquid dinner the night before the test. After midnight, you won't be allowed to eat or drink anything, until the test is complete.

After the test, drink plenty of liquids. You may also need a laxative to help you eliminate the barium. Until the barium's eliminated, your stools will be white.

Lower GI series (barium enema)

Purpose
To examine the large intestine (large bowel) and identify obstructions, tumors, inflammation, or polyps

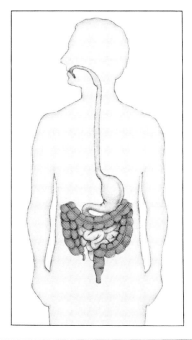

What to tell the patient
The doctor wants to perform an X-ray examination of your large intestine (or large bowel). So that it will show up clearly on X-ray film, your bowel must be as empty as possible.

To help empty the bowel, please drink as much fluid as possible the day before the test. I'll give you oral laxatives and a rectal suppository the night before the test. You'll drink only clear liquids for dinner and won't be allowed to eat or drink anything after midnight.

The test will take place in the X-ray department. First, the doctor will take an X-ray of your bowel to make sure it's completely empty. If it is, he'll position you on your side and prepare to insert a small tube into your rectum. (He may give you medication through an arm vein to relax your bowel, which will make insertion of the tube more comfortable.) After inserting the tube, the doctor will allow a liquid called barium to flow gently through the tube. He may also insert some air through it. Both the barium and the air help your bowel show up better on X-ray film. As he takes the X-ray pictures, the doctor may ask you to change your body position. If you feel the urge to move your bowels during the test, resist this urge by taking slow, deep breaths through your mouth. If the doctor's inserted air through the tube, you may feel some gas pains. Tell the doctor if you become very uncomfortable.

The entire test will take about an hour. Afterwards, you'll be permitted to empty your bowel. Then, you'll wait in the X-ray department while the doctor examines the X-rays. He may decide to take more X-rays before you return to your room.

After the test, I'll give you another laxative to help you eliminate all the barium. Your stools will be white until all the barium's eliminated.

Gallbladder series (cholecystography)

Purpose
To identify gallstones; to diagnose cholecystitis or choledocholithiasis.

Important: Because this test requires ingestion of an iodine dye, it's contraindicated for patients who are allergic to iodine or seafood.

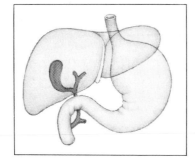

What to tell the patient
Your gallbladder is a muscular pouch located underneath your liver. It stores bile, which is made in the liver and helps you digest fatty foods.

The night before the test, I'll give you some pills called Telepaque* (iopanoic acid tablets). The iodine dye in these pills will concentrate in your gallbladder, causing it to show up clearly on X-ray film. The morning of the test, you may not eat or drink anything until the test is complete.

The test will be performed in the X-ray department and will take about an hour.

Intravenous pyelography (IVP), or excretory urography

Purpose
To assess kidney function and detect obstructions in the urinary tract.

Important: Because this test requires injection of an iodine dye, it's contraindicated for patients who are allergic to iodine or seafood.

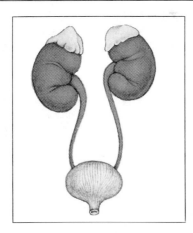

What to tell the patient
The day before your test, drink as much fluid as you can. In the evening, you'll be given only clear liquids for dinner. Then, I'll give you a laxative to clear out your intestinal system so the doctor can clearly see your urinary tract. You won't be allowed to eat or drink anything after that.

The test will take place in the X-ray department. The doctor will ask you to lie down on a table; then, he'll inject an iodine dye into a vein in your arm. You'll experience a warm, flushed sensation, and a metallic or salty taste in your mouth. These sensations will disappear quickly.

When the iodine dye reaches your kidneys, the doctor will begin taking X-rays. Eventually, the dye will flow to your bladder for excretion. Then, he may ask you to empty your bladder, and take more X-rays. The entire test takes 1 to 4 hours.

After the test, please drink as much fluid as you can and ask for some solid foods if you are hungry.

Computerized tomography (CT or CAT scan)

Purpose
To examine cross sections of the brain, liver, lungs, and other internal structures. Some CT scans provide three-dimensional views.

Important: Use of iodine dye during a CT scan is contraindicated for patients who are allergic to iodine or seafood.

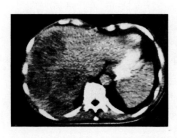

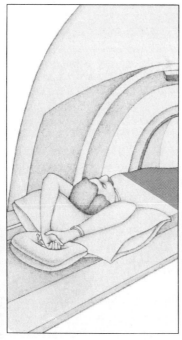

What to tell the patient
The CT scan is an X-ray examination that produces pictures of your internal body structures from all angles. It's completely painless.

You'll go to a special examination room for the test. The doctor or technician will ask you to lie on your back on a table. Because even a slight movement may distort the CT scan, the technician will strap you securely to the table so that you lie as still as possible. Then, the table will carry you through the large, round opening of the CT scanner until the part of your body being X-rayed is inside.

During the test, you'll be alone in the room. However, the technician will watch you from an adjoining room, and you'll be able to talk to him through an intercom, if necessary.

To take pictures of your body from many angles, the CT scanner will rotate around you; you will remain motionless on the table. As the machine rotates, you'll hear clicking sounds. Lie as still as possible. The technician may ask you to hold your breath from time to time. The test will take approximately 15 minutes.

If your patient is to receive a contrast dye, also give him this information: Your doctor's decided to give you an iodine dye, so he can see certain body parts more clearly during this test. The morning of the test, you won't be permitted to eat or drink anything. The doctor may give you the dye before the test (orally or rectally); during the test (by injection into an arm vein); or both. Expect to experience a warm, flushed sensation, and a metallic or salty taste in your mouth after you receive the dye. These sensations will disappear quickly. The entire test will take between 30 to 45 minutes.

Testing

Understanding endoscopy

Endoscopy is a diagnostic procedure that allows the doctor to visually examine a body cavity; for example, a portion of the gastrointestinal (GI) tract or tracheobronchial tree. To perform the procedure, the doctor will use an endoscope.

Most endoscopes are made of flexible plastic, and equipped with a fiberoptic lens. Some are also equipped with cameras, or with instruments that can remove a polyp or obtain tissue samples. The endoscope shown below is designed for anoscopy.

Although you probably won't assist with an endoscopic examination, you're responsible for preparing your patient beforehand, and caring for him afterward. And patient preparation, of course,

includes a clear explanation of what to expect and why the test is needed. For example, tell the patient that he'll go to a special examination room, and that the lights will probably be dimmed to let the doctor see better. If the patient's undergoing bronchoscopy, tell him that the doctor may wear a mask to protect the patient from possible infection. In addition, explain that the doctor may take samples of tissue or secretions during the test for analysis.

Keep in mind that the patient may find these tests uncomfortable, so provide extra emotional support. Answer his questions frankly.

Important: In your hospital, endoscopy may be considered an invasive procedure that requires the patient's written consent.

Test	Tube insertion site	Patient preparation (pre-test)	Patient care (post-test)
Upper GI endoscopy (esophagoscopy, gastroscopy)	Mouth	• Tell the patient that he isn't allowed to eat or drink anything on the morning of the test. Explain that this permits better visualization and minimizes the risk of aspiration. • Tell the patient that he'll receive a local anesthetic (sprayed on his throat), to minimize discomfort while he swallows the tube. • If ordered, give a sedative, such as diazepam (Valium*) 30 minutes before the test. • If applicable, remove the patient's dentures. Report any loose teeth, caps, or bridges that may become dislodged during the procedure. • Report any signs of oral disease; for example, inflammation, bleeding, or sores.	• Provide a quiet, restful environment, if possible. • Position your patient on his side and withhold food and fluid for 2 hours, or until his gag reflex returns. Tell the patient that a side-lying position reduces the risk of breathing saliva into his lungs; ask him to maintain that position until you've determined that his gag reflex has returned. Place a sign over the patient's bed indicating that he's to take nothing by mouth. • Monitor your patient's vital signs for cardiovascular or respiratory complications. Stay alert for bleeding, dysphagia, fever, and neck, chest, or abdominal pain; any of these signs may indicate esophageal, gastric, or duodenal perforation. • After 1 hour, check your patient's gag reflex. To do so, touch the back of his throat with a cotton-tipped applicator or a tongue depressor, using a short, quick motion. If no response occurs, wait 30 minutes and try again. • Unless complications occur, allow your patient to resume his normal diet after the gag reflex returns (usually within 4 hours). Remove the sign from his bed. • Use an analgesic spray to reduce throat soreness. However, don't use a spray that'll impair the patient's gag reflex. • Document all procedures and observations.

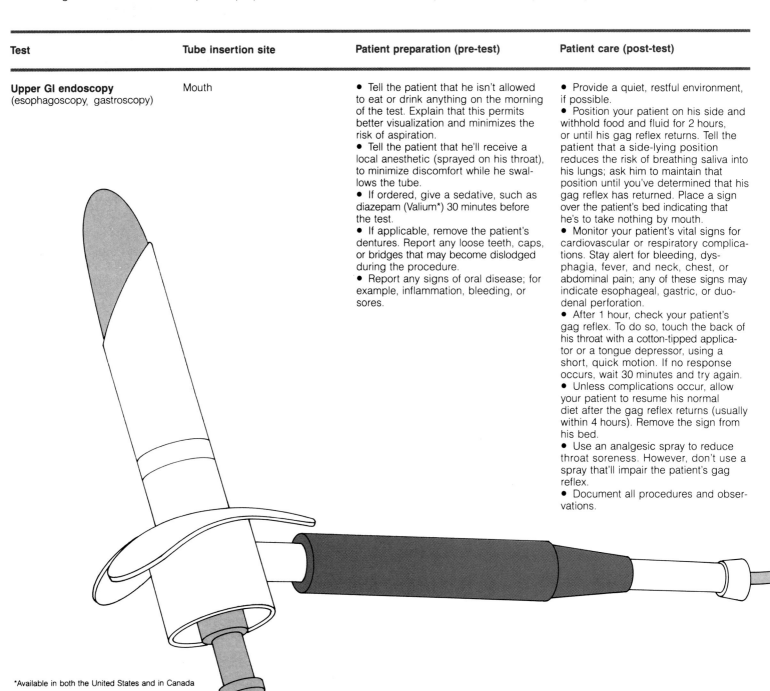

*Available in both the United States and in Canada

Test	Tube insertion site	Patient preparation (pre-test)	Patient care (post-test)
Lower GI endoscopy (anoscopy, sigmoidoscopy or proctoscopy)	Anus	• To help clear the bowel, give the patient a clear liquid diet for 24 hours before the examination. • Give laxatives the night before the test and an enema or suppository the morning of the test, as ordered. *Note:* If the patient has diarrhea or inflammatory bowel syndrome, the doctor will order a low-pressure, tap-water enema. • Alert the patient to the positions he may be asked to assume during the test. For example, explain that he may be asked to lie on his stomach on a special examination table that will elevate his buttocks. Remember, the patient may find this procedure embarrassing as well as uncomfortable, so provide extra emotional support.	• Watch the patient for signs of bowel perforation: bleeding, abdominal distention, or prolonged pain. However, tell the patient to expect some abdominal cramping after the test. • Unless complications occur, the patient may resume normal diet and activities immediately after the test. • Document all procedures and observations.
Tracheobronchial tree endoscopy (bronchoscopy)	Nose or mouth	• Do not permit the patient to eat or drink anything for at least 6 hours before the test. • Instruct the patient to perform thorough mouth care the evening and morning before the test. • To allow better visualization, help the patient perform postural drainage the morning of the test. • Take special care to explain the test, since the patient may find it frightening. Assure him that he'll be given medication to make the procedure more comfortable. Tell him that he'll be positioned on his back. Advise him to relax as much as possible when the tube's inserted, and to breathe slowly and deeply through his mouth, if the doctor inserts the tube in his nose. If the doctor inserts the tube in his mouth, advise him to breathe through his nose. • If ordered, administer atropine sulfate I.M. 30 minutes before the test; this reduces oral and tracheal secretions. Tell the patient that this drug will make his mouth feel dry. • If ordered, administer a short-acting barbiturate 30 to 60 minutes before the test. This sedates the patient, and reduces the stimulating effects of cocaine hydrochloride, the local anesthetic of choice. *Note:* For some patients, the doctor may order a general anesthetic, administered I.V. in the examination room. • Remove the patient's dentures, if he has any. Report any loose teeth, caps, or bridges that may become dislodged if the doctor inserts the tube in the patient's mouth. • Report any signs of oral disease; for example, inflammation or sores.	• Position the patient on his side, or as ordered. If he's conscious, tell him not to attempt swallowing until his gag reflex returns; instead, tell him to let saliva run out the side of his mouth. Provide tissues or an emesis basin. • Watch the patient closely for signs of tracheobronchial trauma or perforation; for example, hypoxia; bleeding, stridor, dyspnea, neck edema, and subcutaneous emphysema around the neck and shoulder. Also, stay alert for cardiac arrhythmias or other signs of myocardial infarction (chest, jaw, or left arm pain; nausea; diaphoresis; cyanosis; dyspnea), which may be caused by vagal stimulation or emotional stress. If you see any of these signs, notify the doctor, and immediately begin support measures. • Post a sign over the patient's bed indicating that he's to take nothing by mouth. • After about 1 hour, test his gag reflex, as described on the opposite page. If no response occurs, wait 30 minutes and try again. • When the gag reflex returns, remove the sign from the patient's bed, and offer him liquids. After 8 hours, he may eat soft foods; unless complications occur, he may resume his normal diet within 24 hours. • If necessary, provide comfort measures for his throat, such as an ice collar. • Encourage deep breathing. • Document all procedures and observations.

Patient teaching

"What will it be like?" If your patient's never had surgery before, he may have a hard time imagining it. In fact, he may feel so uncertain, he'll even hesitate to ask questions. But you can bet he'll be wondering about it. And even if your patient's had surgery before, he's likely to have many of the same fears and questions.

So what's the answer? Patient teaching, of course. In this section, you'll learn what to teach, and why. In addition to preparing your patient and his family for the events and procedures he'll experience, you'll teach him:

• how to deep breathe and cough effectively.

• how to use an incentive spirometer.

• how to participate in intermittent positive pressure breathing (IPPB) therapy, if the doctor considers it necessary.

But what if your patient enters the hospital only one day before surgery? Such a situation leaves little time for patient teaching. To cope with this problem, many hospitals get a head start on patient teaching by sending the patient an informative booklet, along with pre-admission paperwork. Doing so allows the patient to read the booklet at his leisure, and think of questions. If your hospital doesn't distribute such a booklet, consider designing one yourself. Use the information in this section as a guide.

Preoperative teaching: An overview

You want your patient to be fully informed about his planned surgery. At the same time, you realize that he's likely to absorb only a small amount of new information in the short time he's in your care. How can you strike a balance between too much information—and too little?

Concentrate on giving your patient a general overview of his expected surgical experience. Use the information in the following checklist as a guide. Chances are, he'll think of questions as you talk with him. Answer them as completely as possible.

Because most surgical patients spend very little time in the hospital before surgery, we've focused here on the immediate pre- and postoperative period. But if you have contact with the patient before his hospitalization (for example, if you work in a doctor's office), give him additional information about:

• routine preoperative tests; for example, chest X-ray, electrocardiogram (EKG), blood tests, and urinalysis. If your patient's scheduled for elective surgery, he'll probably undergo most of these tests before he enters the hospital.

• using antimicrobial soap. The doctor may ask the patient to begin showering with antimicrobial soap several days before surgery to reduce the risk of wound infection. Repeated use of antimicrobial soap increases its effectiveness at inhibiting bacterial growth on the skin.

• smoking. If your patient smokes, advise him to stop for a minimum of 12 hours before surgery; 24 hours or more is even better. Explain that by doing this, he decreases the risk of postoperative respiratory and circulatory complications.

• valuables. Ask the patient to leave jewelry and valuables home, or arrange to put the items in the hospital safe.

Now, let's consider what to tell the patient about the period *immediately* before and after his surgery. The following information is geared toward the patient who'll undergo elective surgery under general anesthesia. Of course, you'll modify this information, according to your hospital's procedures, the doctor's orders, and your patient's condition.

For convenience, we've presented an overview of the information your patient needs in checklist form. As you see, we've listed events in the order your patient's likely to experience them. But if your patient has any particular questions or concerns, deal with them first. For example, your patient may be most worried about postoperative pain. Discuss his fears with him, and assure him that measures will be available to make him as comfortable as possible. When you've answered all his questions, he'll be more receptive to any other information you feel he needs.

Teaching topic

The day before surgery

☐ Signing a surgical consent form

☐ Preparing the surgical area

☐ Performing additional preop preparation

☐ Attending to preop hygiene

☐ Receiving a sedative (sleeping pill)

☐ Taking nothing by mouth after midnight

The morning of surgery

☐ Attending to preop hygiene

☐ Removing loose objects from the patient's mouth (including dentures and removable caps); removing jewelry (except for a plain wedding band); removing prostheses and other artificial devices or objects (including glasses, artificial eye, and wigs)

☐ Visiting with family

☐ Receiving preanesthetic medication

☐ Arriving at the holding area

☐ Entering the operating room

☐ Waking up in the recovery room

☐ Returning to his room

Additional teaching considerations

• Urge the patient to read the form carefully and ask questions	before he signs it.
• Explain that a large area of skin will be cleaned, and explain why. Tell him when the procedure will take place. • Explain shaving or depilatory hair removal, if hair removal is ordered. • Tell the patient that you'll remove nail polish or artificial	fingernails, if the patient's wearing any, and explain why. • Instruct the patient not to touch the surgical area after it's been cleaned. • Discourage a female patient from performing unnecessary shaving; for example, of her underarms or legs.
• Inform the patient of any additional procedures that the	doctor's ordered; for example, an enema or douche.
• Ask the patient to shower with antimicrobial soap, if ordered, and to shampoo his hair. Remind him to clean his umbilicus. • Encourage him to perform thorough mouth care, including	brushing and flossing his teeth. • Ask him to clean under his fingernails and toenails.
• Explain that this ensures a good night's sleep.	
• Stress that this precaution means that he musn't eat anything (including hard candy), drink anything (including water),	or chew gum. Instruct his family about this, too, especially if they'll be visiting him the morning of the surgery.
• Ask the patient to shower with antimicrobial soap, if ordered, and to perform thorough mouth care. (Remind him not to swallow any water.)	• Ask your male patient to shave, if he's normally clean-shaven (unless his surgery involves his neck or upper chest).
• If appropriate, tell the patient that you'll securely tape his plain wedding band to his finger.	
• Tell the patient that he may visit with his family or speak to them by phone the morning of surgery (according to hospital policy). • Ask his family members to arrive 2 hours before surgery's	scheduled, if they wish to see the patient before surgery. Tell them that they may not be permitted to see him after you've given him preanesthetic medication.
• Explain to the patient that you'll give him a preanesthetic medication after he's completed all preoperative routines, including dressing in a special surgical cap and gown. You'll ask him to urinate before you give the medication. • Explain that after he receives the preanesthetic medication,	you'll raise his side rails and ask him to remain in bed. • Tell him that the medication will help him relax, although he probably won't fall asleep. • Advise him that his mouth will feel dry, since the medication helps dry up secretions.
• Explain that he'll be transported to the operating room's holding area by stretcher. • Warn him that he may have to wait a short time in the holding area until the operating room's ready. Describe the holding	area, and tell him how the doctors and nurses will be dressed. Advise him that the doctors and nurses probably won't talk much to him, to allow the medication to take effect. However, they will observe him closely.
• Explain that he'll be transferred from the stretcher to the operating table. Tell him he'll be securely strapped to the table for his own safety. • Warn him that the operating room may feel cool. Tell him to ask the nurse for another cover, if he's uncomfortable. • Explain that he'll have electrodes applied to his chest, so	the doctor can monitor his heart rate during surgery. • Tell him that the anesthesiologist will insert an I.V. line to administer medication and I.V. fluids during surgery. • Describe the drowsy sensation he'll feel as the anesthesiologist begins giving the anesthetic; urge the patient to concentrate on relaxing.
• Describe the recovery room for the patient. Tell him that the nurse will call his name, ask him to answer questions, and instruct him to do simple exercises, such as wiggling his toes. • Warn him that he may feel some pain at the incision site,	but assure him that the doctors and nurses will take measures, including giving medication (if necessary), to relieve pain. • Describe nasal cannulas and other oxygen delivery systems. Explain that he may have one in place when he awakens.
• Explain that when he's satisfactorily recovered from the anesthetic, he'll return to his room, where he may see his family.	• Warn him that he'll feel drowsy and nap frequently for the rest of the day.

Informing your patient about anesthesia

No matter what kind of surgery your patient needs, he'll require an anesthetic. Make sure your patient understands everything he must know about his anesthetic by following these guidelines:
• Tell the patient the name of his anesthesiologist, and explain that he's a doctor who is specially trained to administer anesthetics. (Of course, if your patient is to be treated by a nurse-anesthetist, you'll explain that she's a specially-trained nurse.) Explain that the anesthesiologist is responsible for his care until he leaves the recovery room.
• Tell the patient that his anesthesiologist will visit him before surgery and answer all of his questions. Encourage the patient to jot down any questions he has beforehand, so he doesn't forget them.
• If your patient prefers one type of anesthetic over another, urge him to discuss this with his anesthesiologist, too.
• If the patient still has questions after talking to his anesthesiologist, try to answer them. If necessary, ask the anesthesiologist to return.

Keep in mind that your patient may have special concerns that he's reluctant to mention. For example, if he's to receive a general anesthetic, he may worry that he'll suddenly awaken in the middle of the operation. Or, he may worry that he'll never awaken at all. Anticipate these concerns by assuring your patient that the anesthesiologist will carefully monitor his condition throughout surgery, so he gets just the right amount of anesthetic—no more, no less.

Your patient may also be concerned about talking while under the effects of anesthesia. If so, explain that he's unlikely to speak coherently while he's unconscious, because of the breathing tube in his throat.

Patient teaching

Preventing respiratory complications

As you know, atelectasis is alveolar collapse. It may affect only a small part of the lung—or, less commonly, the entire lung. Atelectatic alveoli hold no air, which causes them to collapse; as a result, although the alveoli are perfused with oxygenated blood, no exchange of oxygen and carbon dioxide occurs. This condition, called intrapulmonic shunting, causes hypoxia.

Which of your surgical patients risks developing atelectasis? Each one of them. Although some patients are at higher risk than others (see the box at left), *any* patient who fails to expand his alveoli with a deep breath can develop atelectasis—in as short a period as one hour.

An ounce of prevention

With atelectasis, an ounce of prevention's worth a pound of cure. And fortunately, atelectasis *can* be prevented by appropriate nursing measures and careful patient teaching. After surgery, you'll take nursing actions designed to prevent respiratory complications; for example, turning the patient, helping him to ambulate, and percussing his chest to loosen secretions.

But, you'll take action *before* surgery, too. First, you'll tell the patient how postoperative deep breathing and coughing helps speed recovery. Then, you'll teach him postoperative breathing exercises to perform regularly. Finally, you'll oversee his progress throughout recovery.

The most effective exercise for preventing respiratory complications is called sustained maximal inspiration (SMI). SMI produces high negative transpulmonary pressures, which inflate the alveoli to total capacity. In practical terms, SMI is a deep breath that's held for about 3 seconds (the alveolar inflation time), to prevent alveolar collapse. The alveoli then remain inflated for about an hour. So, the postoperative patient should be encouraged to deep breathe at least once an hour.

Teaching deep breathing and coughing

To teach your surgical patient how to deep breathe and cough, use the techniques described in the self-care aids on the following two pages. After explaining each exercise, demonstrate it and ask for return demonstrations. Then, when you're sure the patient has mastered both exercises, give him copies of the self-care aids for reference, and ask him to continue practicing throughout the preoperative period.

However, *don't* teach these exercises if your patient has chronic obstructive pulmonary disease (COPD). Instead, teach him to deep breathe using the exercises on page 37. Then, when teaching him to cough, instruct him to release three short coughs in rapid succession, rather than one vigorous cough. This technique, called *staged coughing,* is less tiring for a COPD patient.

Important: Unless ordered, don't encourage coughing if your patient has had either cataract surgery or a craniotomy.

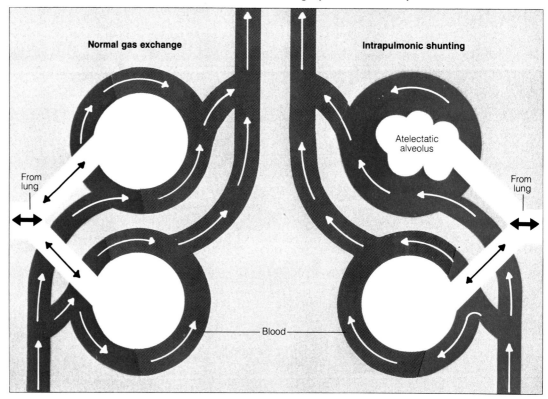

Normal gas exchange   Intrapulmonic shunting

Atelectatic alveolus

From lung   From lung

Blood

Self-care

How to deep breathe

1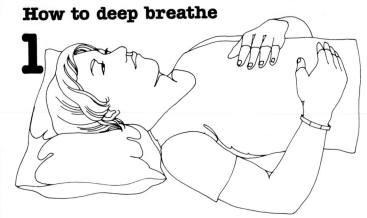

Dear Patient:
After your operation, you'll need to deep breathe several times an hour, to keep your lungs fully expanded. By deep breathing, you'll speed your recovery, and reduce the risk of developing breathing problems as you get well.

To deep breathe correctly, you must use your diaphragm and abdominal muscles—*not* just your chest muscles. This exercise teaches you how. Practice it two or three times a day before surgery. That way, you'll be able to do it more easily after surgery.

Lie on your back in a comfortable position. Place one hand on your chest, and the other over your upper abdomen, as shown here. Flex your knees slightly. Relax.

Exhale normally. Then, close your mouth, and inhale deeply through your nose. As you do, concentrate on feeling your abdomen rising, without expanding your chest. If the hand on your abdomen rises as you inhale, you're breathing correctly.

Hold your breath, and slowly count to five.

2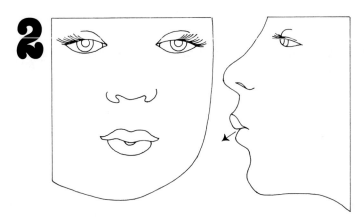

Purse your lips, as though you're about to whistle, and exhale completely through your mouth. (Don't let your cheeks puff out.) Using your abdominal muscles, squeeze all the air out. Your ribs should sink downward and inward.

Rest several seconds; then continue the exercise until you've done it five to ten times.

3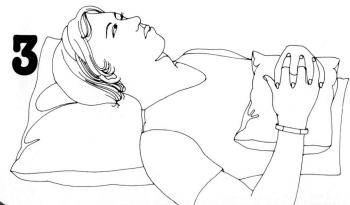

If you're having abdominal surgery, you may be more comfortable if you hold a pillow over your incision, as shown here. Lace your fingers together across the pillow to hold it in place. Then, perform the deep breathing exercise as described above.

Note: You may also perform this exercise while lying on your side, sitting, standing, or as you're turning in bed.

Patient teaching

Self-care

How to cough effectively

Dear Patient:
After your surgery, the nurse will ask you to do coughing exercises at least every 2 hours. Coughing helps keep your lungs free of secretions. You should practice coughing before your surgery, so you can do it easily afterwards. Follow these instructions:

1

Sit on the edge of your bed. If your feet don't touch the floor, the nurse will give you a stool to rest them on. Bend your body slightly forward, as shown here. (After surgery, you may also perform this exercise while lying in a comfortable position, instead of sitting on the edge of the bed.)

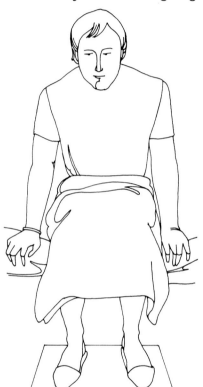

2

Are you having chest or abdominal surgery? Reduce your discomfort while coughing by splinting (supporting) your incision as you cough. To splint your incision, place one hand above the incision and one hand below it, as shown here.

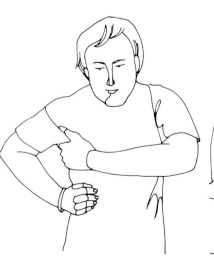

3

If you're lying down, you can splint a chest or abdominal incision by putting a pillow over it, and lacing your fingers together over the pillow.
　Immediately after surgery, you may feel too weak to firmly splint your incision. Don't worry; the nurse will help you.

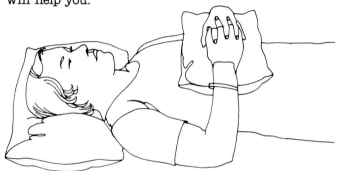

4

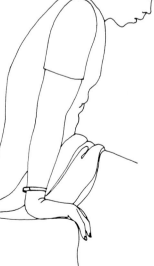

To help stimulate your cough reflex, take a slow, deep breath. Breathe in through your nose, and concentrate on fully expanding your chest. Breathe out through your mouth, and concentrate on feeling your chest sink downward and inward. Then, take a second breath in the same manner.
　Now, take a third deep breath. This time, hold your breath; then, cough vigorously. As you do, concentrate on feeling your diaphragm force out all the air in your chest.
　Repeat this exercise at least one more time.

SPECIAL CONSIDERATIONS

Teaching additional breathing exercises

Does your surgical patient suffer from chronic obstructive pulmonary disease (COPD)? If so, or if he's at high risk of developing postop respiratory complications for any other reason (see the box on page 34), teach him the additional breathing exercises described below. These exercises strengthen the accessory breathing muscles. After surgery, these exercises may also be used along with postural drainage, percussion, and vibration. (For details on performing these techniques, see the last section of this book.)

• Put your patient in a comfortable position; for example, in a semi-Fowler's position with his knees slightly bent at about a 10° angle. As you know, bending the knees decreases tension on the abdominal muscles.

• Firmly place your hands on each side of his lower rib cage, with your little fingers resting on his lowest ribs (see top photo). Encourage him to relax. If he's in a sitting position, ask him to keep his shoulders lowered throughout the exercise.

• Ask him to inhale through his nose, taking a slow, deep breath. As he does so, ask him to expand his lower rib cage outward, against your hands. Urge him not to use his shoulder muscles as he inhales.

• Now, ask him to purse his lips, as though whistling, and to exhale slowly through his mouth. Discourage him from exhaling forcefully, since this may cause his alveoli to collapse, trapping more air in them.

• As he exhales, urge him to concentrate on feeling first his chest, then his lower ribs, sink. As you feel his lower ribs sink inward, gently squeeze his rib cage with your hands to force all the air out from the base of his lungs.

• When he can successfully do this exercise, ask him to practice it with his own hands placed bilaterally alongside his lower rib cage.

• Encourage him to do this exercise for 5 to 10 minutes every hour, or until he becomes tired or short of breath.

Unilateral costal (or segmental) breathing

If your patient's had a lobectomy, or if part of his lung becomes compromised by atelectasis, you'll need to help him improve expansion of the affected area. The following exercise helps.

• Position the patient, as described above.

• Place your hand firmly over the part of the lung that's involved (see bottom photo).

• Ask the patient to take a deep breath through his nose. As he does so, ask him to concentrate on pulling air into the area under your hand, pushing your hand out as he breathes in.

• Then, ask him to exhale slowly, through pursed lips. Instruct him to concentrate on feeling first his chest, and then his lower ribs, sink inward.

• Help the patient to repeat this exercise for 5 to 10 minutes every hour, or until he becomes tired or short of breath.

• Consider teaching the patient how to properly place his hands, in order to do the exercise himself. However, continue to supervise him, to make sure he does the exercise correctly.

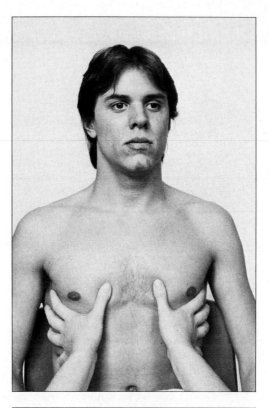

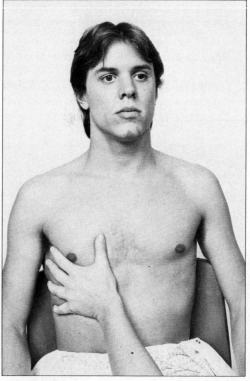

Learning about incentive spirometers

Your patient may understand why deep breathing exercises are important. But after surgery, when he's weak, sedated, or in pain, he may need some encouragement to regularly perform them. Incentive spirometry, which provides instant feedback, may give him the encouragement he needs.

The next few pages show you how to teach your patient about spirometers. But first, consider how they compare.

Spirometers can be divided into two basic types: flow incentive, and volume incentive. A flow incentive spirometer measures the patient's inspiratory effort (flow) in cubic centimeters per second (cc/sec). A volume incentive spirometer goes one step further. From the patient's flow rate, it calculates the *volume* of air the patient inhales. As a result, many volume incentive spirometers are larger, more complex, and more expensive than flow incentive spirometers.

Which type is better for your patient? That depends. For low risk patients, a flow incentive spirometer will probably do the trick. Lightweight and durable, it can be left at the patient's bedside for repeated use, even when you're not there to supervise.

But, if your patient is at high risk of developing atelectasis, you may prefer a volume incentive spirometer. Because it measures lung inflation more precisely, it helps you determine whether your patient is inhaling adequately. And the additional supervision you'll provide when the patient uses this type of incentive spirometer encourages compliance.

Of course, your daily supervision is a must, no matter what type of spirometer your patient uses. Auscultate his lungs before and after he uses the spirometer, and document your findings. This provides a basis for assessing your patient's progress.

Patient teaching

Learning about the Spirocare® volume incentive spirometer

The Spirocare Incentive Breathing Exerciser shown in these photos is an example of a volume incentive spirometer. This lightweight, battery-run device provides immediate feedback to your patient and encourages effective deep breathing. The Spirocare also has a special hold feature that encourages your patient to continue inhaling for several seconds, following the principle of sustained maximal inspiration (SMI). In the following photostory, you'll learn more about the Spirocare's features.

But first, take a look at the chart on the Spirocare's back panel (see the top photo). The doctor (or respiratory therapist) will choose one of the listed volumes as a goal for your patient. Each volume indicates the approximate amount of air your patient inspires when taking a deep breath. As the chart shows, the doctor may choose a volume in the high, medium, or low range.

Depending on the range he chooses, volume goals increase in increments of 125 cc (low range), 250 cc (medium range), and 500 cc (high range). The doctor's choice of range determines how hard your patient must work to achieve a new goal on the volume scale.

As an example, let's compare the low and medium ranges. As you see, a volume goal of 500 cc occurs in both ranges. If the doctor sets a volume goal of 500 cc in the low range, the patient must increase his inspiratory volume by only 125 cc to achieve the next highest goal on the volume scale. But if the doctor chooses the same volume in the *medium* range, the patient must increase his inspiratory volume by 250 cc. The doctor's choice depends on the patient's condition.

Read the photostory to learn how to set up a Spirocare spirometer—and how to teach your patient to use it.

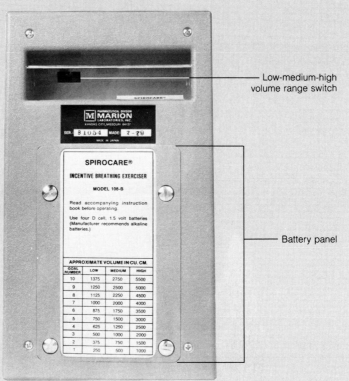

Low-medium-high volume range switch

Battery panel

SPIROCARE®
INCENTIVE BREATHING EXERCISER
MODEL 108-B

Read accompanying instruction book before operating.

Use four D cell, 1.5 volt batteries (Manufacturer recommends alkaline batteries.)

APPROXIMATE VOLUME IN CU. CM.

GOAL NUMBER	LOW	MEDIUM	HIGH
10	1375	2750	5500
9	1250	2500	5000
8	1125	2250	4500
7	1000	2000	4000
6	875	1750	3500
5	750	1500	3000
4	625	1250	2500
3	500	1000	2000
2	375	750	1500
1	250	500	1000

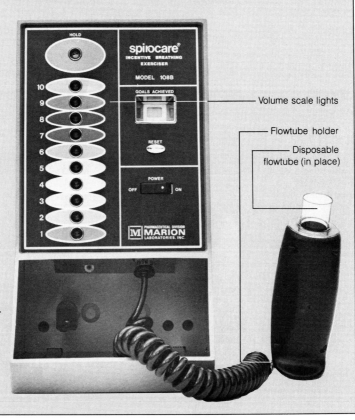

Volume scale lights

Flowtube holder

Disposable flowtube (in place)

Using a Spirocare® spirometer

1 *Your patient, Donald Elliott, is scheduled for gallbladder surgery. He'll need to use an incentive spirometer after surgery to maintain adequate respiratory function. But the time to teach him about the spirometer is before surgery, while he's alert and pain-free. If you're demonstrating the Spirocare Incentive Breathing Exerciser, follow these guidelines:*

Gather the equipment you'll need. In addition to the spirometer and its flowtube (mouthpiece) holder, you'll need a disposable plastic-wrapped flowtube. If the spirometer isn't equipped with batteries, remove the back panel with a screwdriver, and insert four D size batteries. Replace the panel.

Show Mr. Elliott the spirometer, and briefly explain how it works. Tell him that he'll need to use it frequently after surgery to prevent respiratory complications. Encourage him to ask questions.

Press the POWER switch to the ON position.

2 Let's suppose the doctor or respiratory therapist has set a goal of 1500 cc in the medium range. To set this goal, first turn to the spirometer's back panel. Slide the LO-MED-HI volume range switch to the MED (medium) setting.

Before you set the volume goal at 1500 cc, take a look at the chart on the spirometer's back panel. As you can see, 1500 cc is rated number 5 on the medium range scale.

3 Turn back to the front of the spirometer. In the recessed area above the tray, to the right of the flowtube holder's cord attachment, you'll find a black dial. Rotate this dial until a blinking red light appears at 5 on the volume scale.

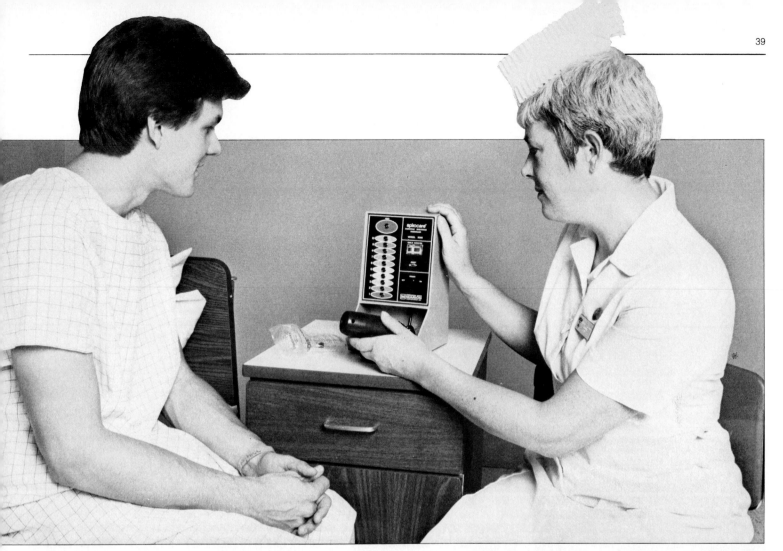

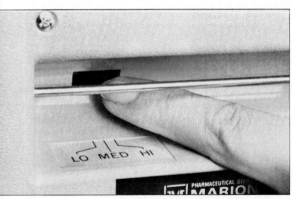

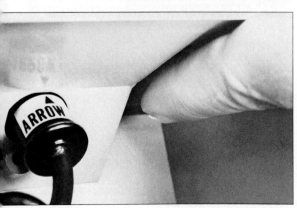

4 Now, pick up the disposable, plastic-wrapped flowtube. Hold the flowtube's shorter flanged end in one hand. To avoid contamination, tear open the plastic wrapper by pushing the flowtube forward, as shown here. As you do so, keep the flanged end wrapped in plastic.

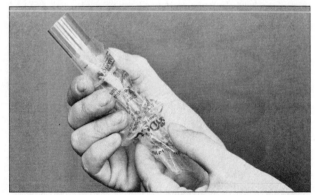

5 Pick up the flowtube holder and insert the exposed end of the flowtube, as the nurse is doing here. With the wrapper still covering the flanged end, rotate the flowtube until its nipple catches in the slot inside the holder. When the flowtube's secure, remove the plastic wrapper, and hand the flowtube holder to Mr. Elliott.

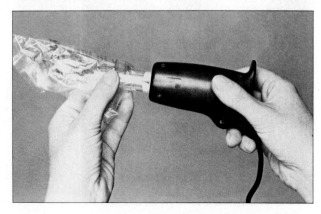

Patient teaching

Using a Spirocare® spirometer continued

6 If necessary, press the RESET button, so the GOALS ACHIEVED window displays 00. Then, take a moment to explain the lights on the front panel. Tell Mr. Elliott that the blinking red light at 5 identifies his inhalation goal. Explain that when he inhales, another red light will appear opposite the number 1, and will begin climbing the scale. If Mr. Elliott reaches his goal, this red light will climb to 5, and the blinking red light at 5 will become constant. If Mr. Elliott surpasses his goal, the constant red light will climb past the blinking light. By watching these lights, he'll receive immediate feedback on how well he did.

Now, point out the HOLD light at the top of the scale. As Mr. Elliott inhales, this light will shine yellow. Ask him to continue inhaling until this light goes out. This helps to fully expand his lungs. Make sure he understands why this is so important.

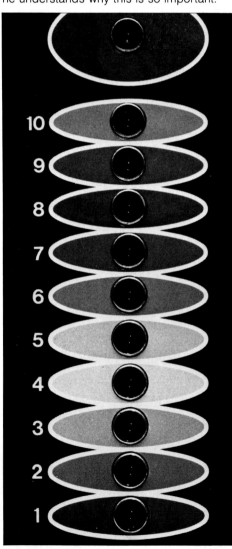

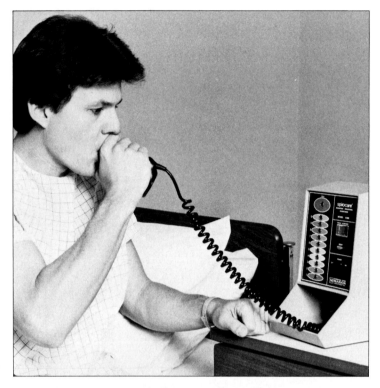

7 Now, Mr. Elliott's ready to use the spirometer. Ask him to firmly wrap his fingers around the flowtube holder and to press his thumb over the flange. Make sure the flowtube's clear and unobstructed. Then, ask Mr. Elliott to place his lips tightly around the flowtube, up to the flange. To perform the deep breathing exercise, instruct him to exhale normally and then to inhale deeply. Ask him to continue to do so until the HOLD light goes out. Then, have him remove the flowtube from his mouth, and exhale normally. Praise him for his effort.

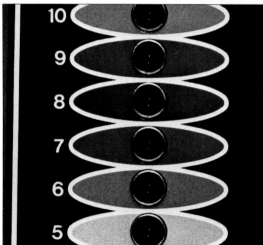

8 Now, point out the GOALS ACHIEVED window to Mr. Elliott. This window will display the number of times Mr. Elliott reaches (or surpasses) his goal. (To keep track of how many times he's achieved his goal each day, instruct him to press the RESET button each morning before beginning his first set of exercises.)

Chances are, the doctor or therapist will want Mr. Elliott to perform this deep breathing exercise five times, at least once an hour. Encourage him to do it more often. As Mr. Elliott becomes stronger, the doctor will set progressively higher goals. *Important:*

Caution the patient to rest as needed between exercises.

Document the date and time of your teaching session, as well as the patient's inhalation volume. Remember, the doctor or therapist may use this preoperative inhalation volume as a baseline reference when setting postoperative goals.

Note: Between exercise sessions, encourage the patient to remove the flowtube, wash and dry it, and store it in a clean plastic bag. Once a day, replace the used flowtube with a clean one. Label the bag with the date you replaced the flowtube.

Using a TriFlo II™ flow incentive spirometer

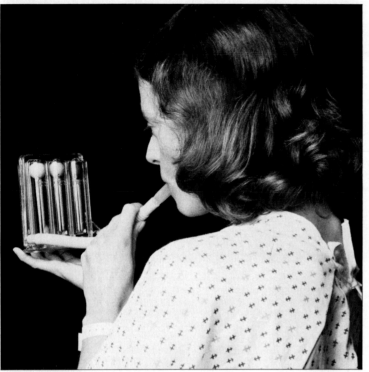

This TriFlo II Incentive Deep-Breathing Exerciser is lightweight, hand-held, and disposable. As this photo shows, it has three separate cylinders, each containing a ball. Each ball, when completely elevated by the patient's inspiration, measures the patient's flow volume as follows: the light blue ball on the left measures 600 cc/sec; the medium blue ball in the middle, 900 cc/sec; and the dark blue ball on the right, 1200 cc/sec.

You'll find the TriFlo II simple to assemble. Just connect the mouthpiece to one end of the tubing, and connect the other end of the tubing to the base of the TriFlo II unit.

Now, you're ready to teach your patient how to use it. Tell her to hold the unit in an upright position, as shown here. (If she tilted it, she'd need less effort to elevate the balls, making the exercise less effective.) Then, ask her to exhale normally, and to place her lips tightly around the mouthpiece.

Let's say the respiratory therapist has instructed your patient to generate a flow rate of 1200 cc/sec. Ask the patient to inhale until all three balls rise to the top of their cylinders, as she's doing in this photo. Then, for maximum alveolar inflation, encourage her to continue inhaling for 3 seconds. If the balls remain elevated for 3 seconds, the patient's doing the exercise correctly.

Then, instruct the patient to remove the unit's mouthpiece from her mouth and exhale normally. Ask her to relax, if necessary, and repeat the exercise as directed by the respiratory therapist.

Ask the patient to remove the mouthpiece after each exercise session, rinse it with water, and dry it. (Of course, if she's on bed rest, you'll do this for her.) Keep the mouthpiece, tubing, and the TriFlo II unit in the plastic bag provided by the manufacturer.

Using a Voldyne® volume incentive spirometer

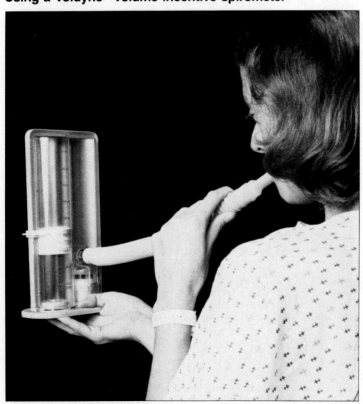

Not all volume incentive spirometers are as complex as the Spirocare (see the information beginning on page 38.) For example, consider the Voldyne Volumetric Exerciser, shown here. Like the TriFlo II, it's lightweight, hand-held, and disposable. The difference? It tells you at a glance the *volume* of air your patient inhales with each effort, rather than the air flow she generates.

To assemble it, attach the mouthpiece to the tubing, and the tubing to the stem on front of the unit.

Next, slide the pointer on the INSPIRED VOLUME cylinder to the volume level prescribed by the doctor or respiratory therapist. As you see here, the nurse has set the pointer at the 1500 ml level. This is the patient's inspiration goal.

Give the exerciser to the patient, and tell her to hold it upright, as she's doing in the photo. Then, instruct her to exhale normally and to place her lips tightly around the mouthpiece. Ask her to inhale slowly until the top of the piston inside the INSPIRED VOLUME cylinder reaches the pointer.

For maximum alveolar inflation, encourage her to continue inhaling for 3 seconds. If she does so correctly, the piston will hover in the cylinder at pointer level. Then, tell the patient to remove the mouthpiece and exhale normally. (The piston will drop.) After the patient rests, ask her to repeat the exercise as directed.

Note: Take a look at the small cup in the right-hand cylinder. If the therapist prescribes deep, *slow* inspiration, the cup should rise only slightly when the patient inhales, so its top is level with the clear, narrow window just below the tubing connector stem.

Ask the patient to remove the mouthpiece after each exercise session, rinse it with water, and dry it. (Of course, if she's on bed rest, you'll do this for her.) Keep the mouthpiece, tubing, and Voldyne exerciser in the plastic bag provided by the manufacturer.

Patient teaching

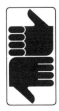

Using intermittent positive pressure breathing (IPPB) therapy

The doctor may want your patient to have IPPB therapy to:
- prevent or treat atelectasis.
- augment bronchodilation.
- deliver deep aerosol therapy.
- loosen secretions.
- ease patient's breathing by reducing $PaCO_2$.

The doctor probably won't order IPPB therapy if your patient has:
- fractured ribs.
- acute pneumothorax or pneumomediastinum.
- subcutaneous or mediastinal emphysema.
- hemoptysis.
- tracheoesophageal fistula.
- pulmonary bullae.
- cardiovascular insufficiency (hypotension, hypovolemia, or arrhythmias).

The doctor may also avoid IPPB treatments if the patient won't comply with treatments, if treatments cause him distress, or if a less complicated therapy will work.

Learning about
intermittent positive pressure breathing (IPPB) therapy

Let's suppose you're caring for 54-year-old Marvin Oblonsky, who's scheduled for a lobectomy. Because he's obese and a heavy smoker, you know he's at high risk of developing atelectasis. And, of course, thoracic surgery adds to the risk.

For a patient like Mr. Oblonsky, the doctor may order IPPB therapy for the first few days after surgery, in addition to deep breathing and coughing exercises. This therapy will help Mr. Oblonsky inflate his lungs while he's too weak to inhale deeply by himself.

How does IPPB therapy work? When the patient inhales through the IPPB machine's mouthpiece, the machine exerts a preset positive pressure, which inflates the patient's lungs. (The machine's airflow stops when the pressure in the patient's mouth reaches the preset pressure.) When the patient exhales, the rapid reduction of pressure loosens secretions and stimulates the cough reflex.

Why isn't IPPB therapy routine? Consider these disadvantages:
- IPPB therapy is less effective at preventing atelectasis than incentive spirometry.
- To ensure that therapy's effective, a nurse and/or specially-trained therapist must supervise every treatment. As a result, IPPB treatment is time-consuming for the hospital staff, and expensive for the patient.
- Prolonged therapy may cause alveolar rupture, resulting in additional cardiopulmonary complications.

For all these reasons, the doctor will want to discontinue IPPB therapy as soon as possible. So, throughout treatment, also encourage your patient to deep breathe, cough, and use an incentive spirometer.

Learn how to operate one type of IPPB equipment by examining the following photograph and text.

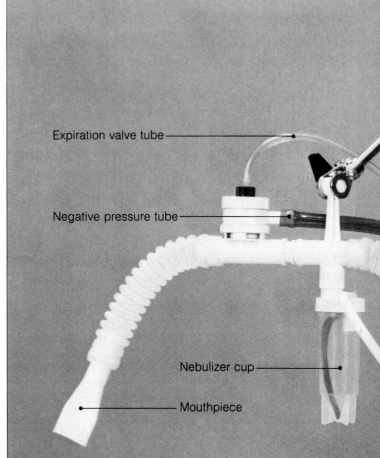

Expiration valve tube

Negative pressure tube

Nebulizer cup

Mouthpiece

The Bennett PR2 respiration unit shown here delivers either intermittent positive pressure breathing (IPPB) therapy, or controlled ventilation to the patient. To prepare the machine for IPPB therapy, follow the steps listed below. *Note:* Your hospital may use a different model of equipment for IPPB therapy. Always check the manufacturer's instructions.
- First, make sure the ventilation rate is turned off. The patient controls the rate during IPPB therapy.
- After attaching the tubing, as shown here, unscrew the nebulizer cup. Place the prescribed medication inside the cup and replace it tightly. *Remember:* Never give a dry treatment; use distilled water to provide humidity if medication isn't ordered.
- Next, connect the pressure hose to the oxygen wall outlet. Turn the pressure control knob clockwise until the gauge reads the ordered pressure. To avoid delivering 100% oxygen, push in the air dilution knob on the machine's side. You'll now get a mixture of air and oxygen.
- Remove the dust cap from the valve. Lift the drum pin, and adjust the inspiration nebulization button on the machine's side until you see a light mist in the nebulizer cup.
- Begin the IPPB treatment as explained in the patient teaching information on the opposite page.

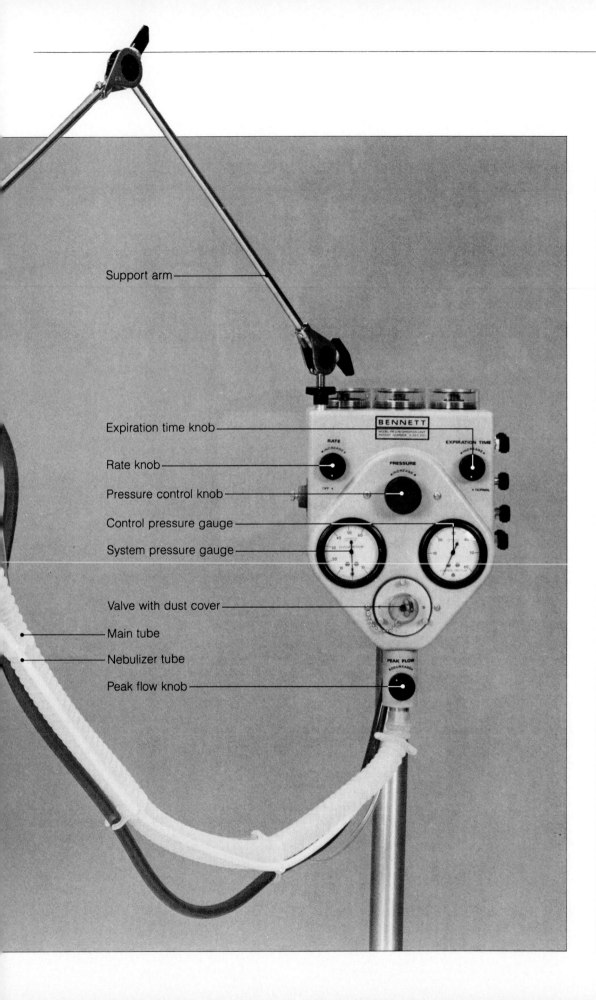

Support arm

Expiration time knob

Rate knob

Pressure control knob

Control pressure gauge

System pressure gauge

Valve with dust cover

Main tube

Nebulizer tube

Peak flow knob

BENNETT

RATE

PRESSURE

EXPIRATION TIME

PEAK FLOW

Preparing your patient for intermittent positive pressure breathing (IPPB) therapy

• Have your patient sit in a chair, with both feet on the floor. If he's on bed rest, place him in a high Fowler's position, or seat him on the edge of the bed, with both feet supported.

• Instruct him to practice breathing slowly and deeply through his mouth. Then, ask him to seal his lips tightly around the mouthpiece. Tell him to inhale slowly, allowing the machine to do the work. When he exhales, have him breathe out around the mouthpiece. Assure him that the treatments will become easier with practice.

As the patient inhales, watch his chest for full expansion. Make sure the patient isn't obstructing the mouthpiece with his tongue.

Nursing tip: If your patient is incorrectly performing the procedure by inhaling through his nose, apply a nose clip.

• Repeat the procedure until the nebulizer cup's empty (usually 15 to 20 minutes). Teach the patient to tap the side of the nebulizer cup periodically so the moisture particles can drop to the bottom.

• After each session, thoroughly wash and dry the mouthpiece, and store it in a clean plastic bag.

Patient teaching

Preparing the family

You know your patient's concerned about his surgery. But others are concerned about it, too—his wife, his sister, his son, and his daughter. In fact, they may be even more worried than the patient himself.

When you prepare your patient for surgery, do you include his family in your plans? You should, because they can be important allies. If they feel as calm and confident as possible, they can provide invaluable emotional support for the patient.

To some extent, your plans depend on your assessment of family dynamics. For example, does the family seem closely-knit and supportive? Or does

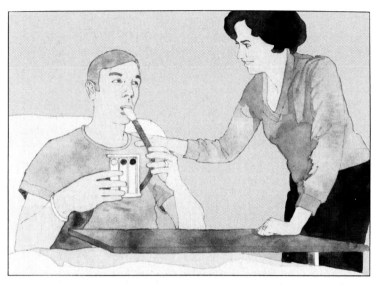

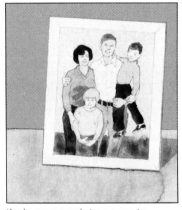

their own anxiety seem to increase the patient's fear? Is the family under additional stress from another source; for example, a recent divorce or death in the family? Do some family members seem to irritate the patient, or make him uncomfortable? All these considerations will affect how much you encourage family members to participate in the patient's care.

But regardless of family dynamics, always take care to inform the family members about all aspects of the patient's hospitalization, including any changes in his condition and care. Remember, his family's under stress, too. They need your support. By making a special effort to keep them informed, you can help them cope. Follow these guidelines:

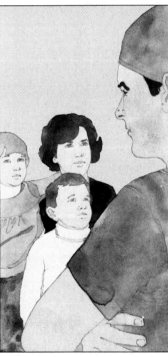

• Include family members in teaching sessions, if possible. For example, help them understand why deep breathing and coughing are important following surgery. After surgery, they can encourage the patient to routinely perform these exercises.
• Inform them of your hospital's visiting policy. Are young children allowed? What are the hours? If your hospital has unrestricted visiting hours, discour-

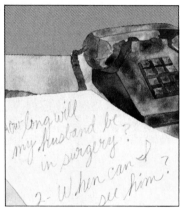

age the family from visiting when routine nursing procedures are scheduled. *Note:* If a family member works during visiting hours, make special arrangements so he can visit when he's able.

After surgery, suggest that only two people visit the patient at once. Remind them that he'll tire easily during recovery.
 Nursing tip: If the family's supportive, suggest that they visit when you're ambulating the patient, and encourage them to help. This way, they can participate in the patient's care.
• Stress the importance of protecting the patient from infection. Tell family members not to visit if they have colds, or feel ill. In addition, remind them not to sit on his bed, since this also increases the risk of infecting the patient. Also,

discourage them from using the patient's bathroom.
• Show family members where to wait while surgery's in progress. If appropriate, tell them the surgeon may meet them there after surgery. Also, assure them that a nurse or receptionist will relay any messages from the surgeon during surgery. In addition, she'll tell them when the patient returns to his room.
• Do family members plan to call your floor for reports on the patient's progress? Suggest that one family member act as a spokesman. Ask that he call you at a convenient time, when you're likely to be free to talk with him. Then, ask him to relay the information to other family members.
 Nursing tip: Consider suggesting a time after the surgeon usually makes his rounds, so you can inform the spokesman of the surgeon's most recent assessment.
• If family members have questions for the surgeon, give them his name and office phone number. Advise them that the surgeon may not be in his office when they call, but that his nurse will tell them when to expect him to call them back. Suggest they jot down their questions, and be near their phone at the time the surgeon makes his calls.
• If family members arrange to meet with the surgeon at the hospital, make sure they tell you or the unit secretary when they've arrived. They should also tell you or the unit secretary if they leave the floor for any reason. This way, you can remind the surgeon that the family's waiting to see him, and ensure that they get together.
• When appropriate, don't hesitate to ask the family members for advice about patient care. For example, ask them how the patient usually copes with stress or pain. Does crying seem to help him? Or does he prefer to remain uncomplaining, no matter what? Their insights can help you tailor your care to the patient's needs.

Procedures

As you know, you must perform a wide range of duties before your patient's ready for surgery. These preoperative procedures include:
• preparing and cleansing the patient's skin.
• following your state's Nurse Practice Act regarding the patient's informed consent.
• applying antiembolism stockings.
• administering preanesthetic medications.
• completing a preoperative checklist.

Whether or not you perform these procedures daily, you can use these pages to refresh and sharpen your skills. We'll explore all these procedures in detail, to help you perform them correctly.

Preparing the skin for surgery

Each person's skin normally harbors all sorts of microorganisms—some harmless, some potentially dangerous. By cleansing the surgical area with an antimicrobial solution or a liquid soap—a procedure commonly called a skin prep—you remove many of these microorganisms, as well as oils and dead skin cells that promote bacterial growth.

No skin prep procedure removes all microorganisms from the skin. But repeated cleansing (using friction) significantly reduces their numbers and inhibits their growth. That's why most preoperative prep procedures follow this pattern:
• For several days before the scheduled surgery, the patient showers regularly with an antimicrobial agent. (If he's scheduled for a craniotomy, he'll shampoo with an antimicrobial agent as well.)
• The night before surgery, the patient shampoos, as well as showers, with an antimicrobial agent.
• The night before surgery, or the morning of surgery (or both), you (or another nurse) will cleanse the surgical area. For most types of surgery, this prep is essentially nonsterile, although you'll observe clean technique as you work. However, for orthopedic surgery, you'll perform one or two sterile preps before surgery, using strict aseptic technique.
• Once the patient is in the operating room, the surgeon will prep the surgical area one more time.

Skin prepping procedures (as well as the specific cleansing solutions used) vary from hospital to hospital. For example, in some hospitals, an orderly or prep nurse performs preoperative skin preps. But in your hospital, you may be expected to perform these procedures for all surgical patients in your care. And these skin preps may include shaving.

To shave, or not to shave?

Traditionally, shaving the surgical area has been standard procedure. And many surgeons still feel that shaving reduces the risk of infection, either from microorganisms on the hair, or from the hair itself falling into the surgical incision. If the patient's hair is unusually thick or coarse, shaving also provides better visibility of the surgical site.

But today, shaving isn't necessarily routine. Because nicks and microabrasions caused by shaving provide a fertile field for bacterial growth, the wound infection rate for patients shaven before surgery is significantly higher than for patients who weren't shaven.

What's the alternative? If your patient doesn't have an allergic sensitivity to depilatories, you may use them to remove hair while avoiding the risk of skin breakage.

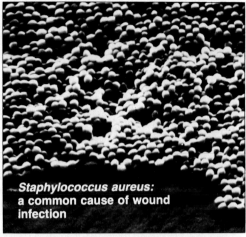
Staphylococcus aureus: a common cause of wound infection

Depilatories remove hair from even hard-to-shave areas (such as the knuckles and ankles), without leaving stubble. But, some authorities believe hair removal isn't necessary unless the patient's hair is very thick or coarse. Long hair may be clipped with scissors or clippers. Thorough prepping cleans the remaining hair, as well as surrounding skin. Nevertheless, many surgeons still order extensive shaving as part of the skin prep.

The wound infection rate rises in proportion to the amount of time between the shave and the surgery. So, if the doctor's ordered a shave along with the prep, perform it as close to the time of surgery as you can—within several hours, if possible. *Note:* If your patient's scheduled for a craniotomy, the doctor will probably shave the patient in the operating room. (Hair removed from the patient's scalp must be saved and is usually put in the hospital safe.)

Locating the skin area to be prepped

How large a skin area should you prep, using these techniques? That depends on hospital policy and the surgeon's preference. Most likely, he'll specify the area. But if he doesn't, consult the guidelines established by your hospital's surgical committee.

As you know, the area to be prepped is much larger than the area of the actual incision. This gives the surgeon the opportunity to make a larger incision, if necessary; it also reduces the risk of contamination of the incision area during draping and other preoperative procedures. Be sure to explain this to your patient as you perform the prep. *Note:* If the perineal area is included in the surgical area, and the doctor's ordered shaving, shave the perineal area last.

To learn the essentials about skin prep procedures, study the information on the following pages. Check your hospital policy for variations.

Procedures

**Performing a nonsterile
shave and skin prep**

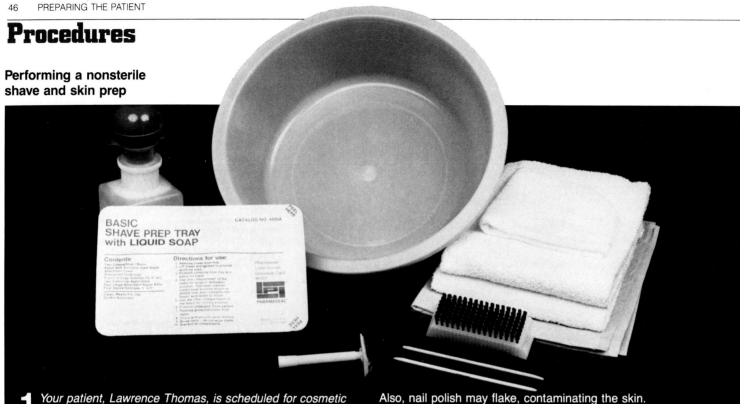

1 *Your patient, Lawrence Thomas, is scheduled for cosmetic
surgery on his right foot. Because Mr. Thomas has heavy,
coarse hair on his legs, the doctor has ordered his lower right
leg (from just above the knee to the foot) to be shaved as well
as cleansed. Since his surgery's scheduled for 9 a.m., you'll
perform the prep in the morning at about 6 a.m. This way, you'll
be able to complete the prepping procedure before it's time to
give him his preanesthetic medication. Remember: By shaving the
patient the morning of surgery, rather than the night before,
you significantly reduce the risk of infection.*

In the following photostory, you'll see how to perform the skin
prepping procedure. As you work, remember to observe clean
technique. *Note:* Never wear nail polish when you do a skin prep,
because small cracks in the polish can harbor microorganisms.

Also, nail polish may flake, contaminating the skin.

Obtain a disposable skin prep kit, which contains: a disposable
razor (with blade), gauze sponges, cotton balls, cotton-tipped
applicators, liquid soap, a double-compartment basin, and disposable towels for draping. You'll also need an extra razor (with
blade), warm water, bulb syringe, clean towels and a washcloth,
a bed-saver pad, orangewood sticks, a large basin, and a hand
or nail brush. In addition, obtain a gooseneck lamp. And if the
doctor's ordered an antimicrobial prep, you'll need the antimicrobial
solution he's ordered.

For some patients, you may also need scissors to clip long
hair and fingernails, and nail polish solvent to remove nail polish.
(Remember, during surgery, the doctor will periodically check
the patient's nailbeds for signs of cyanosis.)

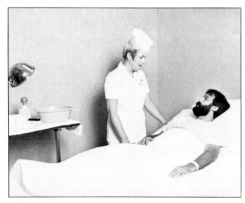

2 Explain the procedure to the patient,
and answer his questions. Explain why
preparing such a large skin area is necessary, so he doesn't become unnecessarily
frightened. Then, position him comfortably,
so the area you'll prep is easily accessible.

Thoroughly wash your hands, paying
particular attention to your fingernails. Remove all finger jewelry.

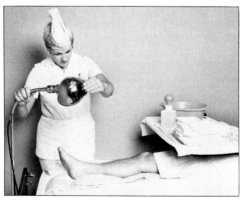

3 Drape Mr. Thomas' leg with a towel, so
the area to be prepped is exposed.
Place the bed-saver pad under his leg.
Then, position the gooseneck lamp so the
area is well-lighted.

Closely examine his leg for broken skin or
skin eruptions. If you see any, report them
to the doctor before proceeding, and
document your observations.

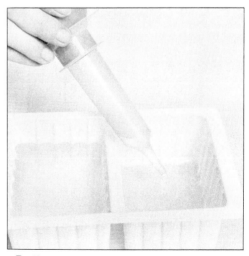

4 Pour warm water into one side of the
disposable basin. Pour the liquid soap
into the other side of the basin, and dilute
with water, as shown here. Now, you're
ready to begin cleansing the skin.

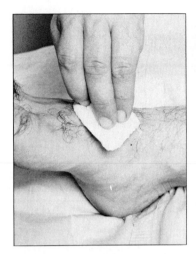

5 Moisten a gauze sponge in the water; then, in the liquid soap. Using a circular motion that creates friction, use the sponge to create lather on the patient's foot. (Friction helps dislodge microbes on the skin.) Work from the proposed incision site outward, to avoid contaminating cleansed areas.

For Mr. Thomas, you'll begin at his foot and work up his leg. This sequence also provides a longer period for his foot to soak in the lather you create. Soaking helps to soften the hair, which reduces the risk of skin abrasions when you shave.

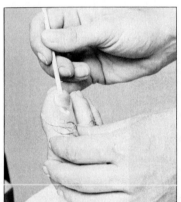

6 When you've lathered Mr. Thomas' leg to above his knee, allow it to soak in the lather. While you wait, use an orangewood stick to clean under Mr. Thomas' toenails. Then, use the brush to scrub calluses and nailbeds.

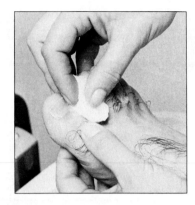

7 Next, use a sponge or cotton-tipped applicator to scrub the creases between his toes. Remember to create friction as you do so.

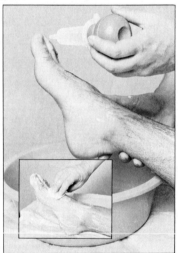

8 To remove the contaminants you've loosened with the brush and orangewood stick, rinse Mr. Thomas' foot. Support it over the large basin, as the nurse is doing here. Then, use the bulb syringe to gently squirt warm water over his foot.

[Inset] Relather his foot, as necessary. Now, you're ready to shave his leg and foot.

Important: If the soap on his leg has become dry, relather his leg before you shave.

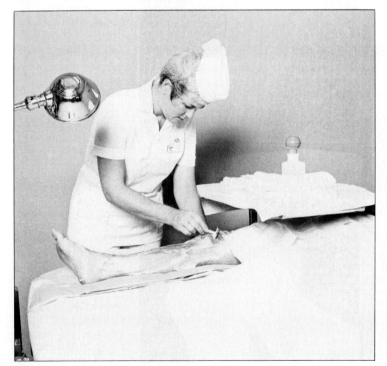

9 First, gently stabilize the patient's skin with your nondominant hand, as shown here. (However, don't pull the skin taut.) Then, beginning slightly above the knee, shave the hair in the direction it grows. Use short, gentle strokes. Continue shaving down his leg, toward his toes, working from the anterior to the posterior side. Take care not to nick the skin. Remember, a close shave isn't necessary. The soap will clean the stubble as well as the skin.

As you work, periodically clean the razor, as necessary, by swishing it in the basin of water. Discard the razor if the blade becomes dull, and continue shaving with the extra razor. To avoid skin irritation, rinse excess soap off the skin you've shaved, and thoroughly dry the skin.

When you finish the procedure, closely examine the shaved skin. Note skin abrasions, nicks, or cuts caused by shaving. If you see any, document them and report them to the doctor.

Ask the patient to take a shower, if possible, using antimicrobial soap. If the patient can't shower for any reason, carefully rinse all hair clippings and excess soap from his skin.

Wrap used materials in the bed-saver pad, and dispose of them according to your hospital's infection control standards. Discard the used razors in an appropriate container for sharp objects.

Supply the patient with a clean gown. Make him comfortable, and stress the importance of keeping the prepped area clean until surgery. Thoroughly wash and dry your hands. Finally, document the entire procedure. If hospital policy requires it, complete an incident report describing any skin nicks or eruptions you may have caused in the surgical area.

Procedures

How to apply sterile gloves

1 *Whenever you perform a sterile orthopedic prep and wrap, you'll need to apply sterile gloves. Do you know how to apply sterile gloves following strict aseptic technique? If you're not sure, read these guidelines:*

Begin by removing all jewelry from your wrists and fingers. However, if you're wearing a plain wedding ring, you may keep it on. Wash your hands thoroughly and dry them with a paper towel.

Then, open the package containing the gloves, as shown here. As you do, take care to touch only the top edges of the package.

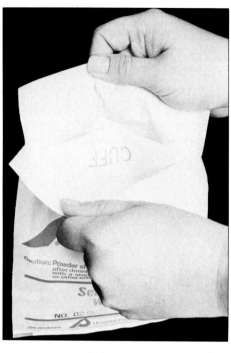

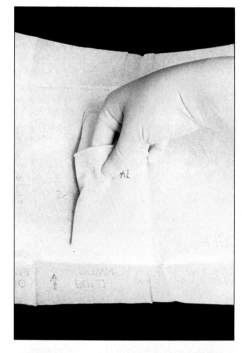

4 Slip the fingers of your gloved hand under the cuff of your left glove, as shown in this photo.

2 Maintaining aseptic technique, open the package's inner wrap. Grasp the folded edge of the right glove's cuff with your left hand, as the nurse is doing here.

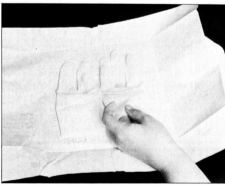
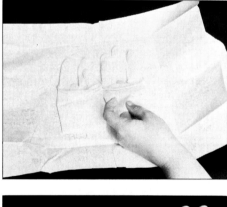

5 As you insert your left hand into the glove, pull the glove on with your right hand. To avoid contamination, be sure your gloved right hand touches only under the cuff of the left glove.

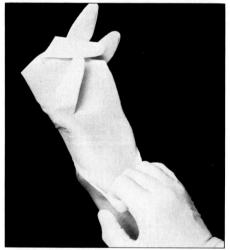

3 Next, slip your right hand inside the glove. Avoid touching the outside of the glove with the fingers of your left hand. If your fingers do touch the outside of the glove, consider it contaminated. Discard the glove, obtain a new package of sterile gloves, and begin the procedure again.

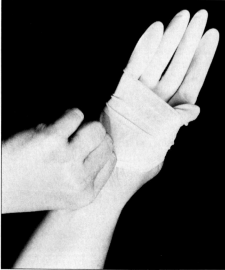

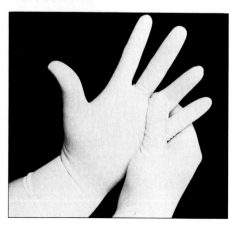

6 Now, adjust both gloves so they fit properly. Check to be sure no gaps exist between your fingertips and the ends of the gloves. (If necessary, obtain smaller gloves, and repeat the procedure.) Inspect the gloves for nicks or tears. If you see any, also obtain a new pair of sterile gloves.

Performing a sterile orthopedic prep and wrap

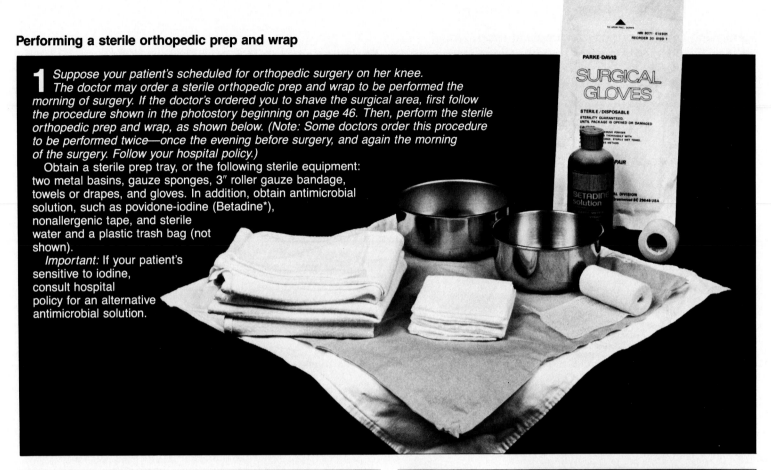

1 *Suppose your patient's scheduled for orthopedic surgery on her knee.*
The doctor may order a sterile orthopedic prep and wrap to be performed the morning of surgery. If the doctor's ordered you to shave the surgical area, first follow the procedure shown in the photostory beginning on page 46. Then, perform the sterile orthopedic prep and wrap, as shown below. (Note: Some doctors order this procedure to be performed twice—once the evening before surgery, and again the morning of the surgery. Follow your hospital policy.)

Obtain a sterile prep tray, or the following sterile equipment: two metal basins, gauze sponges, 3″ roller gauze bandage, towels or drapes, and gloves. In addition, obtain antimicrobial solution, such as povidone-iodine (Betadine*), nonallergenic tape, and sterile water and a plastic trash bag (not shown).

Important: If your patient's sensitive to iodine, consult hospital policy for an alternative antimicrobial solution.

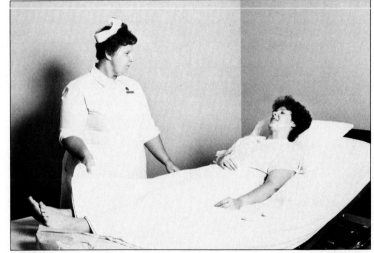

2 Open the plastic trash bag, and place it near your working area. You'll use it to dispose of used sponges.

Explain the procedure to the patient. Tell her that the surgical area will remain wrapped until surgery, to keep it as clean as possible. (If the doctor's ordered a second prep before surgery, be sure to inform the patient.)

Next, wash your hands thoroughly. Using strict aseptic technique, create a sterile field by placing a sterile towel or drape on a clean, dry surface. (If you're working with a sterile tray, use the tray's outer wrapping.) Unwrap all sterile equipment and drop it on the sterile field.

*Available in both the United States and in Canada

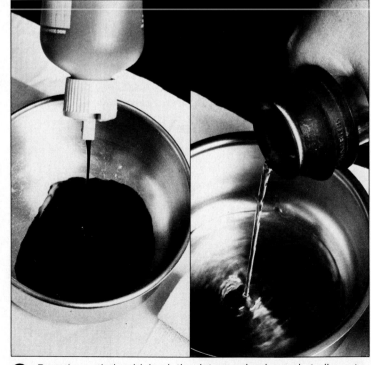

3 Pour the antimicrobial solution into one basin, and sterile water into the other. Take care not to contaminate the sterile field by splashing liquid.

Procedures

Performing a sterile orthopedic prep and wrap continued

4 Grasp a sterile drape by its edges and ask your patient to raise the leg you'll be prepping. Then, place the sterile drape under it, as shown here. Ask the patient to lower her leg on the drape.

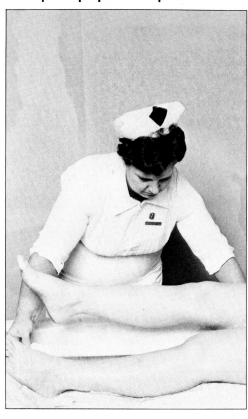

6 Dip a sterile sponge in the antimicrobial solution. Using a circular motion, begin to scrub the patient's knee. Start at the proposed incision site and work outward. Remember to create friction as you work. After 3 minutes, discard the sponge and continue scrubbing with a clean one. Repeat this procedure (using a clean sponge every 3 minutes) until you've scrubbed the surgical area for a total of 10 minutes.

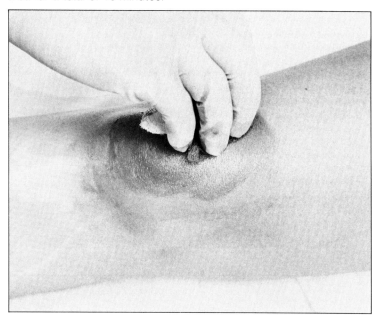

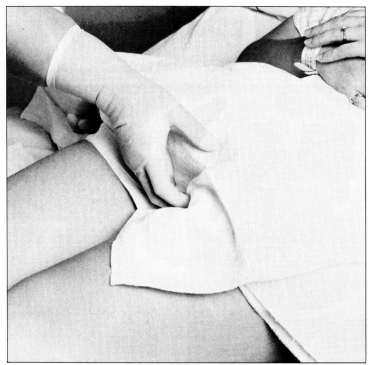

5 Put on sterile gloves, as shown in the preceeding photostory. Then, drape the patient to expose her leg. Keep the rest of her body covered.

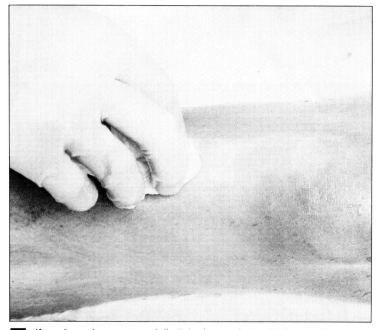

7 If you're using a potentially-irritating antimicrobial scrub (instead of an antimicrobial solution), or if the orthopedic wrap will be in place overnight, reduce the risk of skin irritation by rinsing the patient's leg with sterile water. To do so, dip a gauze sponge in the sterile water, and gently wash the skin you've just cleansed. Then, to prevent chapping, dry the skin with another sterile sponge.

8 To keep the skin as clean as possible, apply a sterile wrap. Use a sterile drape or towel to cover the surgical area.

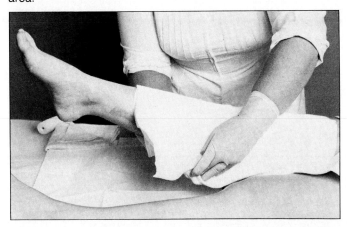

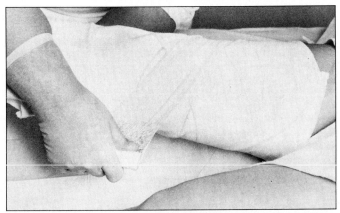

9 Fasten the wrap securely with 3" roller gauze, as shown here. Or, use nonallergenic tape instead.

10 Remove your gloves. Dispose of the gloves and all other disposable equipment, according to your hospital's infection control standards. Thoroughly wash and dry your hands. *Important:* Ask the patient to tell you if her prepped skin begins to feel itchy or irritated. If it does, remove the sterile wrap at once. Quickly assess the patient's skin, and notify the doctor.

Finally, document the entire procedure in your nurses' notes.

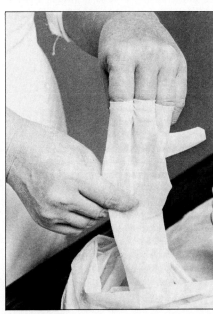

Using a depilatory

Let's say the doctor expects you to use a depilatory cream to remove the hair from your patient's hand. Before you begin, take these important steps.

First, gather this equipment: depilatory cream, applicator stick or tongue depressor, bed-saver pad, disposable gloves, tissues, washcloth, and towels.

Then, inspect the surgical area for rashes, irritation, inflammation, or broken skin. Don't apply the cream if you see any of these conditions. Instead, notify the doctor.

Next, test the cream on the patient's skin. To do so, apply the cream to a small area of skin (about 1" square) that's distant from the surgical area. (A fairly sensitive area, such as the patient's inner arm, is a good choice.) Wait about 20 minutes. *Important:* If the patient complains of a burning sensation, remove the cream immediately.

After 20 minutes, remove the cream and inspect the skin. If the skin appears normal, prepare to apply the cream to the surgical area. However, if the skin seems irritated, notify the doctor before proceeding.

Read any special directions for the cream you plan to use. Then, follow these general steps:
• Place a bed-saver pad under the surgical area to protect the bed linens. Explain the procedure to the patient. Tell him why hair removal's necessary.
• Put on disposable gloves.
• Apply a thick layer of cream over the surgical area, spreading it evenly against the direction of hair growth. Make sure the cream touches the skin at every point. *Important:* Always keep the cream away from the patient's eyes and mucous membranes. If the cream touches these areas, immediately flush with water.
• Leave the cream on for about 15 minutes. Then, remove the cream by *gently* scraping the skin with an applicator stick or tongue depressor (against the direction of hair growth), as the nurse is doing in the photo below. As you do, take care not to abrade the patient's skin. Wipe off the applicator stick or tongue depressor with tissues, and dispose of the tissues. Continue this procedure until you've removed most of the cream.
• Finally, thoroughly rinse away the remaining cream, and pat the area dry with a towel. (If your patient's fair-skinned or allergy-prone, minimize the risk of skin irritation by applying a neutralizing solution, such as dilute acetic or boric acid, after removing the cream. Pat the skin dry.)
• Wrap the applicator stick or tongue depressor inside the bed-saver pad, and discard the pad, according to your hospital's infection control standards.

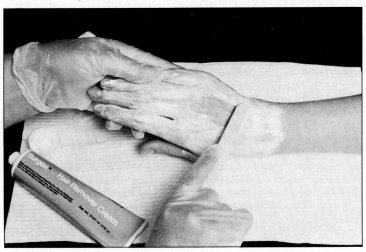

Procedures

Obtaining informed consent

Each patient must sign a consent form before undergoing surgery. The signed form protects the hospital, staff, and doctor from certain legal claims by the patient or his family; and the patient from having any procedure performed without his knowledge.

The doctor is responsible for explaining to the patient what surgical procedure will be performed, the possible complications of surgery, the alternatives to surgery, and the probable postoperative effects. By signing the form, the patient states that the doctor has explained that information to him, and that the patient understands it.

The law varies from state to state as to who can obtain consent from the patient. In some states, the doctor is required to obtain the patient's signature on a consent form; in others, the nurse may get it instead. *Important:* Make sure you know exactly how your state's Nurse Practice Act defines your responsibilities. Follow those guidelines, no matter what your hospital's policy is.

If your state's Nurse Practice Act permits you to obtain the patient's consent, your duties include:
• making sure the patient signs the consent form before being given any medication, including preanesthetic medication, that may cloud his ability to think. The patient's consent is not legally valid if he signs after receiving any such medication.
• asking the patient if the doctor has thoroughly explained the procedure and its implications to him.
• asking the patient if he fully understands the procedure and has no questions.
• filling out the consent form and explaining each part to the patient.
• witnessing the patient's signature on the form.
• recording in your nurses' notes the patient's response to your questions, and the date and time he signed the form.

If you suspect that the patient doesn't fully understand the procedure to be performed, or has doubts about the procedure, notify the doctor. Record in your nurses' notes the time you did this.

Suppose your patient can't read the consent form or sign his own name for some reason (for example, he's illiterate, or a quadraplegic). Ask two people, or as many as your hospital requires, to witness his mark on the form (or his signal of consent). Then, document exactly what's taken place, including the names of all witnesses, in your nurses' notes.

If the patient can't give consent because of physical reasons (for example, he's in a coma) or for legal reasons (he's a minor), then try to obtain consent from the patient's spouse, father, mother, eldest child, or legal guardian. But keep in mind that an emancipated minor is allowed to give his own consent to medical and surgical procedures. (An emancipated minor is someone who hasn't reached the legal adult age but is totally self-supporting. However, interpretation of this definition may vary from state to state.) *Note:* If you have any doubt about who has the authority to give consent, call the hospital's legal department.

If the patient refuses to sign the consent form, or decides against having surgery after signing it, don't try to change his mind. Instead, notify the doctor immediately, and document the circumstances.

Learning about antiembolism stockings

As you know, antiembolism stockings help prevent blood clot formation in a patient whose mobility is restricted. This preventive function is essential, because thrombophlebitis or phlebothrombosis can lead to potentially fatal pulmonary embolism. Pulmonary embolism alone causes a large proportion of all deaths from postoperative complications.

How do antiembolism stockings work? By compressing the capillaries and small veins of the patient's legs. Doing so forces blood into large veins, accelerating the flow so the blood can't pool and clot.

For optimum benefit, the stockings must fit correctly. If they're too tight, they could restrict the patient's circulation, encouraging blood clot development, rather than correcting it. If they're too loose, they'll have no effect. So, measure your patient very carefully. We provide general measuring and application instructions in the following photostories. But, keep in mind that measurements, application, and care methods vary from brand to brand. Always follow the specific instructions from the manufacturer.

Most surgical patients will wear these stockings into the operating room. Afterward, they'll wear them for as long as mobility is restricted, or as the doctor orders. However, don't put the stockings on a patient who:
• has just undergone vein ligation.
• has a circulatory problem such as severe arteriosclerosis, ischemia, vascular disease, or edema from congestive heart failure.
• has a leg disorder or deformity (unless ordered).

How do you care for a patient wearing antiembolism stockings? Remove the stockings every 8 hours and leave them off for at least 1 hour.
✆ *Nursing tip:* Consider removing the patient's stockings before his daily bath, during ambulation, or when he's dangling his legs over the edge of the bed.

After removing the stockings, wash and dry your patient's legs. (If you apply a powder or lotion, do so without vigorously massaging the patient's legs or feet.) Then, assess the entire leg for circulation, sensation, and skin integrity. Also, examine the skin between his toes for any developing pressure sores.

Note: Instruct your patient to check his calf frequently for redness, swelling, or tenderness. If your patient's stockings have toe holes, instruct him to also do frequent quick peripheral circulation checks.

If your circulatory assessment reveals decreased or absent pedal pulses, dusky-colored toenail beds, or reddened areas, first make sure the stockings fit correctly. If they do, notify the doctor. The patient may have a circulatory problem. Also, notify the doctor if the patient complains of leg pain. Document your findings in your nurses' notes.

Measuring for antiembolism stockings

1 *Suppose the doctor's ordered antiembolism stockings for your patient. To obtain the correct size stocking, measure your patient accurately. Here's how:*

First, position your patient lying on her back or side. If she's just been walking, or sitting with her legs in a dependent position, elevate her lower legs and feet for 5 to 10 minutes. This position assists venous return and reduces leg vein engorgement so you can obtain accurate measurements.

Note: When you elevate her legs, avoid applying pressure beneath her knees.

2 Now, position your patient's legs flat on the bed. To fit knee-length stockings, measure the largest part of her calf, as shown.

3 Then, position the patient on her side. Measure from the back of her knee to the bottom of her heel.

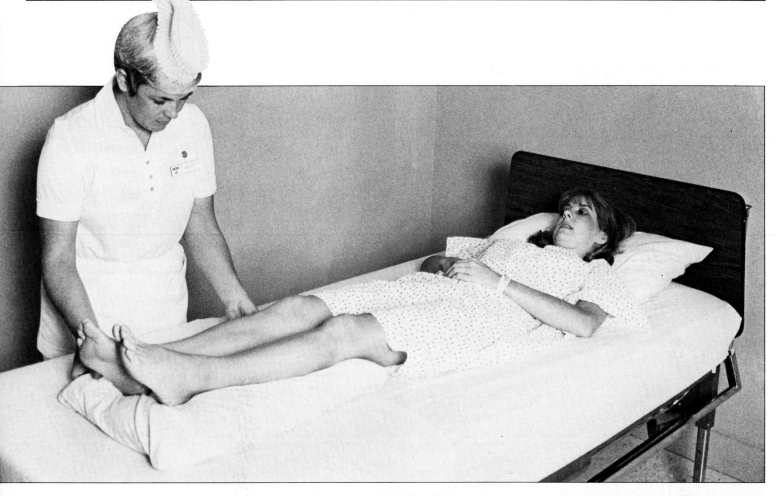

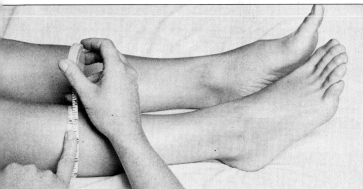

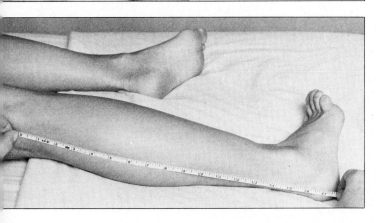

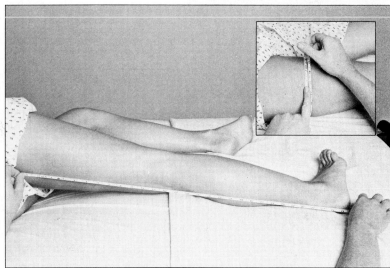

4 Has the doctor ordered thigh- or waist-length stockings? If so, first measure the largest part of her calf, as shown in frame 2. Then, position the patient on her side and measure from her gluteal furrow down to her ankle.

Then, measure the largest part of her thigh (see inset).

Establish baseline measurements for your patient by noting them in her care plan. Then, to obtain the correct stocking size, compare the patient's measurements with those in the table given on the stocking package.

Note: Is your patient obese, very thin, or long-legged? You may have to obtain a special size stocking from an orthopedic supply store.

Procedures

Applying antiembolism stockings

1 *Apply whatever length antiembolism stockings your patient needs shortly before she's scheduled to receive preanesthetic medication.*

Just before you apply them, recheck the circulation in her legs. To do this, note their color, appearance, and temperature. Also, check the patient's pedal and popliteal pulses, bilaterally. If her legs appear cool or cyanotic, or if you detect unequal pedal pulses, notify the doctor before proceeding.

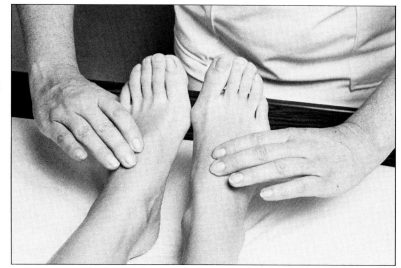

2 To apply the stockings, turn one stocking leg inside out. Then, slip your hand into the stocking up to its heel. Grasp the center of the heel and turn the stocking's foot right side out as far as the heel. Centering the patient's heel in the stocking heel band, place the stocking foot over her foot, as shown here.

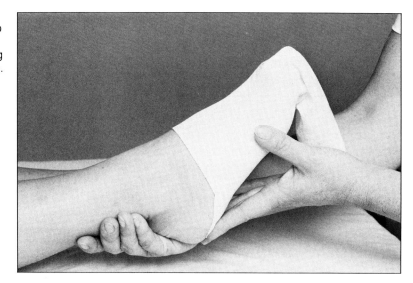

3 Gather the rest of the stocking in your hands and fit it *smoothly* over the rest of her leg.

Note: Avoid wrinkling the stockings. Wrinkles create pressure points and can impair local skin circulation.

Repeat steps 2 and 3 for the patient's other leg.

If you're applying waist-length stockings, make sure you fit your patient with an adjustable belt. Check to be sure the belt's waistband or side panels don't press against any external devices, such as a catheter. Attach the stockings to the belt.

When both stockings are properly applied, elevate both legs above the patient's heart level. Doing so helps prevent blood stasis and clotting.

Postoperatively, instruct your patient to elevate her legs after she walks, dangles her legs over the edge of the bed, or sits in a chair.

Important: When your patient sits or dangles her legs, make sure she doesn't apply pressure on her popliteal spaces.

Encourage the patient to periodically flex and extend her feet and legs, and to regularly rotate her feet in a circular motion.

Document the procedure in your nurses' notes.

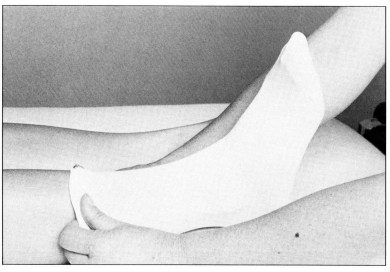

Learning about preanesthetic medications

How much do you know about preanesthetic medications? No doubt you're aware of the four types: sedatives and hypnotics; tranquilizers; narcotic analgesics; and cholinergic blockers. You probably also know that the specific medication and dosage ordered by the doctor depends on your patient's condition, age, and the type of anesthetic he'll be receiving during surgery.

But do you know why the doctor may order a sedative instead of a tranquilizer? Or what preanesthetic medication causes urinary retention or hesitancy? Study the chart below to learn more about preanesthetic medications. *Important:* For complete details on specific types of preanesthetic medications, refer to the NURSING DRUG HANDBOOK™ or the NURSE'S GUIDE TO DRUGS™.

Before administering *any* preanesthetic medication, remember these important guidelines:
- Plan to administer preanesthetic medication parenterally, 1 to 2 hours before surgery, as ordered.
- Double-check drug, dosage, route, time, and patient identity.
- Check the patient's blood pressure.
- Make sure the patient has urinated.
- After administering the medication, raise the bed's side rails. Create a relaxing atmosphere by darkening the room and ensuring quiet.
- If the patient has cigarettes or cigars, remove them from his reach and once again instruct him not to smoke.
- Document the steps you've followed in your nurses' notes.

Sedatives and hypnotics
For example: pentobarbital sodium (Nembutal Sodium*)
Advantages
- Reduces anxiety
- Reduces amount of general anesthetic needed during surgery
- Provides preoperative sedation

Disadvantages
- Decreases the patient's blood pressure and pulse
- May alter the patient's temperature regulatory mechanism
- Depresses central nervous system (CNS). Possible side effects include drowsiness, sleep, or coma.
- May cause respiratory depression

Cholinergic blockers (parasympatholytics)
For example: atropine sulfate, scopolamine hydrobromide
Advantages
- Reduces body secretions; for example, gastric acid, saliva, perspiration, and tracheobronchial mucus

Disadvantages
- May cause restlessness and confusion
- May cause urinary retention and hesitancy
- Interrupts vagal impulses, which may cause tachycardia
- Drying of body secretions may lead to thick mucus congestion in lungs.

Tranquilizers
For example: chlorpromazine hydrochloride (Thorazine) or diazepam (Valium*)
Advantages
- Reduces anxiety
- Relaxes skeletal muscles
- Some (for example, diazepam) produce anticonvulsant effects

Disadvantages
- May cause dangerous hypotension during and after surgery
- May cause confusion, drowsiness, diminished reflexes, mental depression, or coma

---

Narcotic analgesics
For example: meperidine hydrochloride (Demerol*) or morphine sulfate*
Advantages
- Provides preoperative sedation when the patient's in pain
- Reduces pain and anxiety by interfering with central nervous system pain conduction, and altering the patient's emotional response to pain
- Reduces amount of anesthetic needed during surgery

Disadvantages
- May induce nausea and vomiting
- May cause respiratory depression, progressing to Cheyne-Stokes respiratory pattern
- May cause postural hypotension

*Available in both the United States and in Canada

Using a preop checklist

Before your patient leaves his room for surgery, make sure all preoperative routines and procedures are completed. Avoid overlooking anything by using a checklist like the one below.

As you perform each procedure on the list (or confirm that a procedure's been completed), check it off by signing your initials. If another health care professional is performing some of the procedures, ask him to check them off by signing his initials also. *Important:* Make sure all test results are documented before you check off a test as completed. Notify the doctor of any abnormalities.

When the patient goes to the operating room, send the checklist with him. An operating room nurse in the holding area will double-check each item before the patient enters the operating room area.

Patient's name *Marian Welsh*
Room *403ᴬ* Date *11/21/81*

ID band	✓	LK JD
History and physical	✓	LK
Doctors' consultations	✓	LK
Consent form	✓	LK
Blood T/C	✓	LK
CBC	✓	LK
U/A	✓	LK
Chest X-ray	✓	LK
EKG	✓	LK
Special tests	Upper GI	LK
NPO after midnight	✓	LK
Prep	LK	✓ 11/21 6 a.m.
Vital signs	LK	130/84 – 76 – 18 T-98
Dentures	none	LK
Prostheses	none	LK
Jewelry	ring taped	LK
Makeup, nails	✓	LK
Cap and gown	✓	LK
Voided	✓ LK	JD
Preanesthetic medication	✓	JD

Drugs and dosages *Nembutal 50mg I.M., Demerol 50mg I.M. – Atropine 0.4mg I.M.*
Time medicated *8:15 a.m.*

By whom *Joyce Doebler, RN*
Unit nurse *Linda Kratz, RN*

Operating room nurse _____

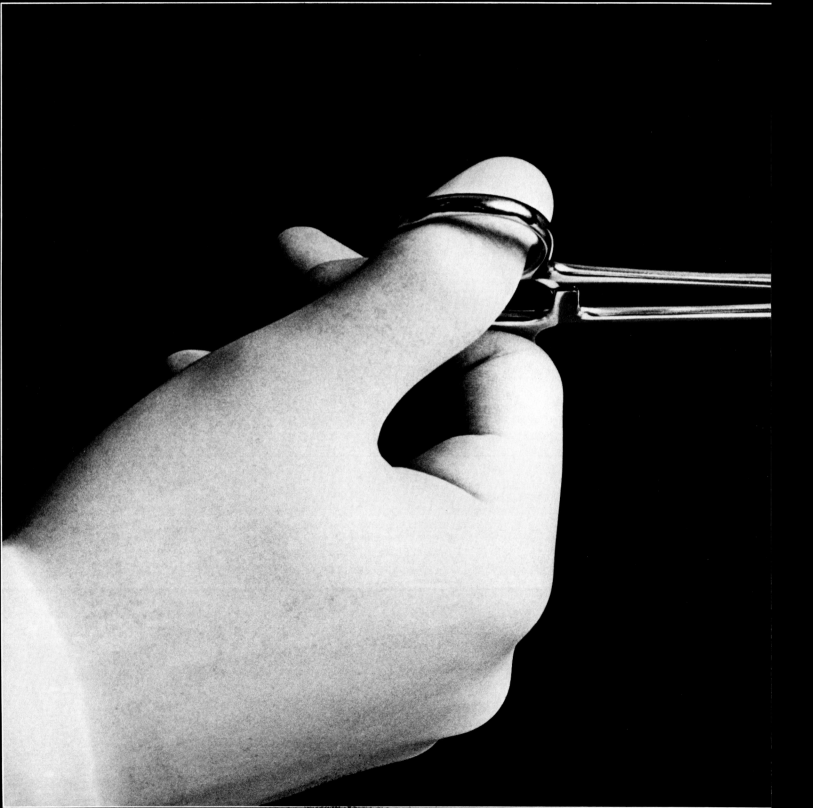

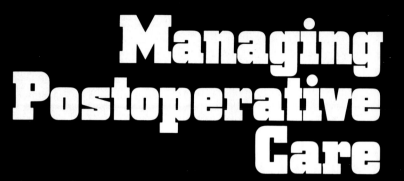

Managing Postoperative Care

Immediate care
Pain management
Ongoing care

Immediate care

Your patient's recovery from surgery depends to a large extent on the quality of care he receives postoperatively. Whether you work in your hospital's recovery room or a medical/surgical unit, you'll need to know the latest techniques and procedures for immediate postop care.

To update your knowledge of the basics—and provide you with helpful tips from experienced nurses—we suggest you read the following pages carefully. In them, you'll learn:
• how to assess your patient's condition following surgery.
• how to monitor the recovery of a patient who's received a spinal anesthetic.
• how to cope with your patient's pain in the recovery room.
• how to prepare your patient's room for his return from the recovery room.
• how to safely transfer your patient from stretcher to bed.

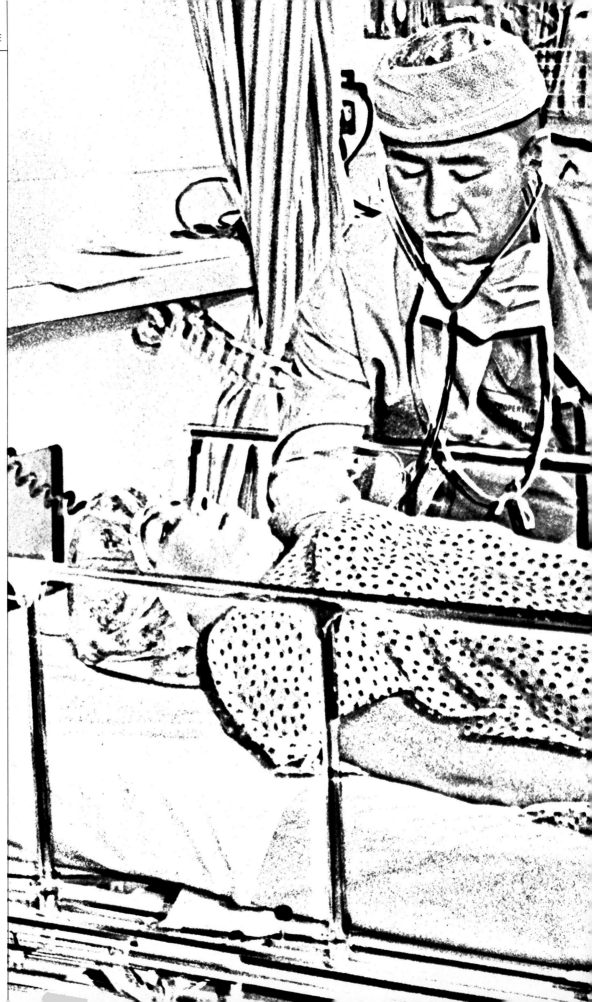

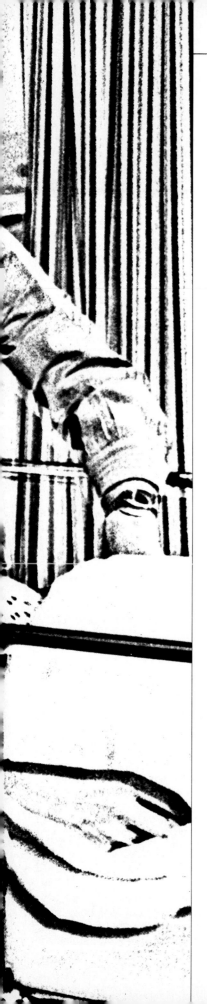

Caring for a patient in the recovery room

Clara Rawling, a 34-year-old travel agent, has just undergone a hysterectomy. She's still unconscious from the anesthetic, thiopental sodium (Pentothal sodium*), and she has an oropharyngeal airway in place to keep her airway open.

As you know, Mrs. Rawling will proceed directly from the operating room to the recovery room where she'll remain until the anesthetic's effects have greatly diminished.

If you're the nurse on duty in the recovery room, you'll receive the following information from Mrs. Rawling's anesthesiologist:
• type of surgery performed
• muscle relaxants, narcotics, anesthetics, and any other medications administered prior to and during surgery
• patient's vital signs
• any problems (such as hemorrhage) encountered during surgery
• presence of an I.V. line, the type of solution being infused, and the rate of infusion
• presence of drains or other aids, such as catheters
• preexisting conditions, such as a cardiac problem, that might have implications for the immediate postop period
• immediate postop instructions regarding anesthetic effects.

Document this information carefully on the recovery room admission note. Then, keep it in mind as you assess your patient's postoperative status. Perform your assessment as soon as your patient arrives in the recovery room, using the chart on the following pages as a model.

This initial assessment provides the baseline information against which you'll compare all subsequent recovery room assessments (done every 15 minutes). Between your assessments, check your patient's vital signs every 5 to 10 minutes.

Does your assessment reveal that your patient's in pain? Read the text on page 62 to find out what to do.

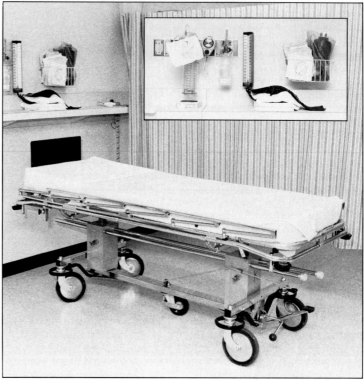

*Available in both the United States and in Canada

Note: When your patient recovers consciousness, she may have questions about her surgery's outcome. Be prepared to supply accurate information. If necessary, consult with her surgeon.

Releasing a patient from the recovery room

Is your patient ready to leave the recovery room? Only the anesthesiologist can release the patient. But, you'll assess the patient and notify the anesthesiologist when you think she's ready. Consider this possible if she's easily awakened, alert, and oriented, her airway remains open without an artificial airway, and her vital signs are stable. Many patients achieve this status within their first postoperative hour.

Some hospitals employ a scoring system to determine whether the patient's ready to leave the recovery room. Under such a system, you rate the patient on each major assessment area, such as cardiovascular status or respiratory status. When she accumulates a certain total number of points across all areas (7 out of 10, for example), the anesthesiologist may release her to a nursing unit.

When you've been ordered to release the patient, call the nurse who'll receive the patient on the nursing unit. Give her the latest information about the patient's condition, including vital signs, consciousness level, and general condition.

But, suppose the patient's condition doesn't stabilize. For example, what if she begins bleeding from separated sutures? Notify the surgeon, who may return her to the operating room for suture reinforcement. What if the patient remains unconscious? Notify the anesthesiologist. The patient may be experiencing a reaction to the anesthetic, or may be hypoxic. Suppose the patient's fully awake but her vital signs are unstable, or she manifests cardiac irregularities. Notify her anesthesiologist. The patient may require transfer to the intensive care unit for further observation.

Immediate care

Nurses' guide to postoperative assessment

When assessing Mrs. Rawling's postop condition, you'll evaluate all her body systems. But, of course, some aspects of your assessment are more immediately critical than others. For example, you'll check your patient's blood pressure before you check her peristaltic function, to make sure she isn't developing signs of shock.

So, when you perform your assessment, we recommend that you proceed in the order indicated on these pages. But, whether you follow this sequence or a slightly different one, try to stick to the same order for each subsequent assessment. If you're consistent, you're less likely to overlook a crucial step.

Also, continue to observe your patient closely, even when you're not performing a formal assessment procedure. Watch for *any* change in your patient's status, whether it's an obvious skin color change, or a more subtle indicator such as mild confusion. Take advantage of every opportunity for observation; for example, during your patient's transfer from the recovery room stretcher to her bed. And, always focus on your *whole* patient—don't concentrate solely on her vital signs, or on the particular care you're giving her at the moment.

Remember to document all your findings. Compare your findings with the preoperative and operating room assessment measurements. Report any significant changes to the doctor immediately.

Cardiovascular system
● Take your patient's blood pressure. Immediately compare it with her preoperative and operating room measurements. Increased blood pressure may indicate pain. Decreased blood pressure may indicate shock, hemorrhage, or oversedation. *Note:* If a patient was hypertensive before surgery, any decrease in postoperative blood pressure might indicate a

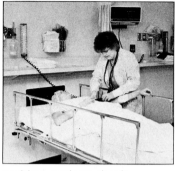

problem such as shock.

Suppose you find a significant difference between her current and previous blood pressure measurements. Check the blood pressure in her other arm. If the pressure in the opposite arm is close to her previous measurements, use that arm for all subsequent measurements. But if a significant difference remains, notify the doctor.
● Determine the rate, rhythm, and quality of your patient's pulse by taking an apical pulse for 1 minute. Auscultating for 1 minute helps you to detect any cardiac arrhythmias. Compare pulse rate, rhythm, and quality with previously-recorded values. An increased pulse rate could indicate shock, hemorrhage, hyperthermia, or pain. A decreased pulse rate could indicate respiratory problems, increased intracranial pressure, or spinal shock. Obtain a radial pulse rate also, and compare it with the apical rate. Report any difference between the two pulse rates to the doctor.
● Observe the patient's skin for color, temperature, and moisture. Note especially her lips and nailbeds. To check her peripheral circulation and tissue perfusion, assess capillary filling by pressing on her fingernail beds. They should blanch; then flush rapidly. Also, check to make sure pedal pulses are present and equal bilaterally. Perform a bilateral assessment of any other peripheral pulses that are distal to a dressing or cast.
● Obtain an oral temperature if the patient can cooperate, or if the surgical procedure per-

mits. Otherwise, take a rectal temperature. A slight temperature elevation is common postoperatively, but you should bring to the doctor's attention any temperature higher than 101° F. (38.3° C.). An elevated temperature in the first few postoperative days may indicate dehydration, or complications such as atelectasis or a respiratory infection. (After 3 days or so, it may indicate a wound infection.)

Respiratory system
● Observe your patient's respirations for rate, rhythm, and depth. Remember, oversedation from pain medication or a general anesthetic can cause respiratory depression.
● Observe her chest for symmetrical movement. Check to see if the patient uses any accessory muscles during respiration. Excessive use of accessory muscles and chest asymmetry are early signs of respiratory difficulty. These signs may appear before visible changes in the patient's respiratory rate, rhythm, and depth.
Note: Use of accessory muscles and chest asymmetry may also indicate a preexisting condition, such as chronic obstructive pulmonary disease.
● Cup your hand and briefly hold it palm down over the patient's nose and mouth to estimate the volume exhaled. She should exhale enough air to inflate a plastic sandwich bag (300 to 400 ml).
● Suppose choking respirations or inadequate exhaled volume indicate that your patient's airway is obstructed. Try to open

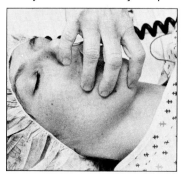

her air passages by repositioning her head and neck, unless contraindicated. Hyperextend her neck and position her head in midline position, without a pillow. If she has no artificial airway in place, insert an oropharyngeal airway. If she has an endotracheal tube in place, check to see if she's biting down on it. (Inserting an oropharyngeal airway as a bite block will correct this problem.) If none of these measures works, begin nasotracheal suctioning to remove excess secretions.
● Auscultate breath sounds in both lungs and compare them. Diminished or absent breath sounds in one lung (accompanied by chest asymmetry) may indicate a pneumothorax. Or, if your patient has an endotracheal tube in place, it may have slipped into her right main bronchus, blocking the left main bronchus. If so, you'll hear diminished or absent breath sounds and see chest asymmetry on her left side.
● If your patient has an endotracheal tube in place, make sure she meets the following criteria before you remove it: her vital signs are stable; she can lift her head off the pillow for a few seconds; she is breathing a sufficient volume of air (300 to 400 ml); and she has regained her gag, cough, and swallow reflexes.

Neurologic system
● Assess your patient's level of consciousness. To do so, call her name to see if you're able to arouse her easily. If not, try to wake her by gently touching her. If she remains unconscious, observe for muscular irritability or restlessness.
● If she's conscious, ask her to push out her oropharyngeal airway. Then, determine her orientation to person, place, and time. Do so by asking her simple questions such as, "What's your name?", "Where are you?" and "What day is it?"
● Evaluate general motor ability in all her extremities. Perform antigravity tests to

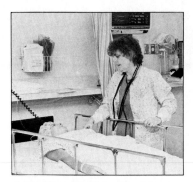

determine whether she has equal strength bilaterally. Have her lift her legs about 6 inches off the bed. Push down on both her legs, while she tries to resist that pressure. Perform the same test on her arms.
• If your patient says she's in pain, assess her pain. (See the guidelines on page 70.)

Wound dressing
• Check the dressing to see that it's dry and intact. *Important:* If you can't readily see the dressing, temporarily reposition the patient.
• Note the presence of any bleeding or drainage. Does the patient have a Penrose drain in place? This could account for any heavy drainage. Use a marking pen to encircle the stained area of the dressing. Initial the circle and note the date and time. Check the dressing every 15 minutes for as long as you see wound drainage on the dressing. If you see unexplained heavy drainage, or any bright red bleeding, notify the doctor immediately. Document the color, odor, and estimated amount of any drainage, each time you check it.
• Don't change a postoperative

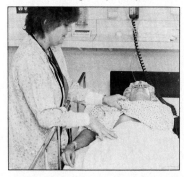

dressing unless the doctor's order specifically instructs, or unless the dressing's been dislodged. Do reinforce the dressing if drainage soaks through it. But, don't reinforce it more than once without notifying the doctor.
    In most cases, the doctor does the first postoperative dressing change. Doing so enables him to assess the condition of the wound, as well as to remove any packing or drains.

Gastrointestinal system
• Auscultate the patient's abdomen for bowel sounds, which indicate peristaltic activity. General anesthetics, abdominal surgery, and narcotics usually decrease intestinal peristalsis for about 24 hours. A return to normal peristaltic function is indicated by 5 to 35 rumbling and gurgling sounds per minute, with loud, prolonged gurgles over the large intestine. As you know, normal peristaltic sounds must be present before the patient eats or drinks anything. Otherwise, she may vomit.
    Note: Medication, patient movement, or obstruction (such as bowel obstruction, or an obstructed nasogastric tube) may also cause nausea and vomiting. If your patient has a nasogastric tube in place, check its patency at least once every 2 hours.
• If the patient vomits, turn her on her side and suction out any remaining vomitus in her mouth, nose, and trachea. Note its amount, color and consistency. Record on the intake and output sheet the amount of vomitus. Remember to check the nasogastric tube for correct placement. It may have been dislodged when the patient vomited.
• Observe and palpate the patient's abdomen to detect distension or tenderness. Rigid distension with tenderness may indicate gastrointestinal tract dysfunction or intraabdominal hemorrhage. With abdominal surgery, rigid distension

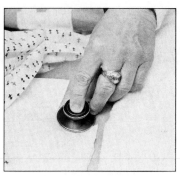

may also be a response to pain and tenderness. (Soft distension may accompany obesity.)

Genitourinary system
• Observe, palpate, and percuss the patient's abdomen for any bladder distension from urinary retention. Start at the symphysis pubis and move upward. Both the anesthetic and the trauma of manipulation during surgery can cause urinary retention. To prevent fluid overload, monitor output.
• If your patient has an indwelling (Foley) catheter in place, she should produce a continuous flow of urine at a rate of 20 to 30 ml per hour. Notify the doctor if her output is less than 20 ml per hour.
• If your patient doesn't have an indwelling catheter in place, record her first urination. This should occur within 8 hours postoperatively. Note the time, and the amount, color, and odor of the urine. Enter the amount on the intake and output record. *Note:* If the surgical procedure involved the urinary tract or the uterus, the urine may be bloody for 12 to 24 hours.
    Important: If the patient doesn't urinate within 8 hours,

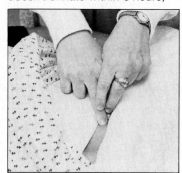

the doctor may order straight catheterization.

Equipment (I.V. lines and drainage devices)
• Locate and identify all drainage systems the patient has in place. If the patient has a drainage system in place, identify the drainage source (bladder or chest, for example.) If the patient has several tubes in the surgical incision, label each tube according to origin; for example, jejunum and stomach. Check all tubes for patency.
• If ordered, connect the drainage tube to a drainage container or suction device.
• Record the amount of drainage present. Enter the amount on the patient's intake and output record. Then, compare it with any previous records.
• Note the location and appearance of the I.V. insertion site. Look for signs of inflammation or infiltration such as redness, warmth or coolness, and swelling. Also, check the I.V. line for patency.
• Make sure the I.V. site dressing is labeled with the date and time of I.V. insertion, as well as the type and size of needle or catheter used.
• Check the fluid being infused as well as any added medication, to make sure it conforms to doctor's orders. To prevent fluid overload, closely monitor the amount of fluid infused (in addition to urine and drainage output). If the patient has an infusion pump, check it to make sure that the flow rate is set as ordered and the machine's infusing the solution at the preset rate.

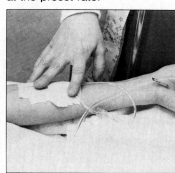

Immediate care

Learning about spinal anesthesia

Has your patient received a spinal anesthetic rather than a general anesthetic? As you know, when the doctor administers a spinal anesthestic (also known as subarachnoid block or SAB), he's injecting a drug such as procaine hydrochloride (Novocain*), tetracaine hydrochloride (Pontocaine*), or lidocaine hydrochloride (Xylocaine Hydrochloride*) directly into the spine's subarachnoid space. When the drug takes effect, it blocks spinal nerve transmission. Depending on the dose and injection site, the doctor can selectively block the sympathetic, sensory, motor, or proprioceptive modalities of the patient's nervous system—without inducing unconsciousness.

However, because a spinal anesthetic blocks spinal nerve transmission, it can also cause complications and side effects. In the operating room, the primary complication that can be caused by this type of anesthetic is a total spinal block. This complication compromises the patient's ability to breathe because his diaphragm and intercostal muscles are paralyzed. His blood pressure may also drop, because of vasomotor paralysis. If this condition is not treated within 3 minutes, the patient will suffer possibly-fatal brain damage.

Sooner or later, you may be responsible for monitoring a patient recovering from a spinal anesthetic. Do you know what to do? Or what side effects to expect? For starters, carry out the cardiovascular and respiratory assessments we recommend for the patient who's received a general anesthetic (see pages 60 and 61).

To assess the neurologic status of your patient recovering from a spinal anesthetic, have him wiggle his toes. If he can, you'll know

that some of the sympathetic nerve blockage has dissipated. When your patient regains both motor ability and sensation in his legs and toes, you'll know he's fully recovered from the anesthetic. But, keep in mind that full recovery may take up to 12 hours. And, although this complication is rare, a patient who's received a spinal anesthetic may never regain motor ability or sensation in his legs.

Here are some common side effects of spinal anesthetics, and how to deal with them:
• *Headache* is usually caused by decreased cerebrospinal fluid (CSF) pressure caused by CSF leakage from the puncture site. Help your patient by positioning him flat on his back and keeping him quiet. Provide plenty of fluids; about 3,000 ml daily, as ordered. Also, encourage him to turn from side to side without raising his head. For a severe headache, the doctor may order aspirin, with or without codeine.
• *Backache* may be caused by paraspinal muscle paralysis. (These muscles maintain normal spinal curvature.) To help your patient, place a pillow in the small of his back.
• *Arachnoiditis* usually results from infection or chemical irritation caused during spinal anesthetic administration. To help your patient, administer antibiotics, and provide about 3,000 ml of fluid daily, as ordered.

Note: For most patients, arachnoiditis can be prevented by following strict aseptic technique and administering proper anesthetic concentrations.

When caring for your patient, remember to document everything in your nurses' notes.

MINI-ASSESSMENT

Coping with your recovery room patient's pain

Your patient's just waking up from the anesthetic. Groggily, he tells you he's in pain. What's your response? First, you'll assess his pain to determine both its origin and severity.

To assess his pain, follow the guidelines on page 70. Remember, your patient's level of consciousness might limit your assessment. Perhaps he can't answer probing questions about his pain. Even so, you must try to define his pain as precisely as you can.

Surgical incising, retracting, and suturing probably cause most of his pain. This type of pain usually requires treatment with an analgesic. But, perhaps your patient's pain is caused by a distended bladder or tight dressings. Or, maybe he's improperly positioned, which places stress on his suture line. You can easily correct any of these problems without resorting to an analgesic. Also, a patient may have throat discomfort after endotracheal tube removal. You can relieve this problem with an anesthetic spray. However, never use one that will impair his gag reflex.

On the other hand, some nonsurgical cause may account for the pain. You can easily mistake anginal chest pain for incisional pain in a patient who has had thoracic or abdominal surgery. So, don't jump to conclusions in assessing your patient's pain. Be sure to notify the

patient's attending doctor immediately if your patient experiences pain that is not associated with the surgical procedure.

When to give pain medication
Whether or not you give pain medication in the recovery room depends on your hospital's policy. But most hospitals do require you to notify the anesthesiologist if, based on your assessment, you think your patient needs medication. The anesthesiologist can then decide whether to medicate the patient or release him immediately to the nursing unit. In one hospital, the anesthesiologist might order a partial dose of analgesic for the patient, and then release him to the nursing unit. (A full dose could oversedate the patient, and possibly cause circulatory or respiratory depression.) Another hospital might require the patient to remain in the recovery room under observation for an additional hour after receiving pain medication. A third hospital might encourage the anesthesiologist to release the patient from the recovery room as soon as the patient's condition stabilizes, without medicating him.

The general trend today is to avoid medicating the patient in the recovery room. But, if your hospital does permit giving pain medication there, see page 72 for information on how to administer it.

---

*Available in both the United States and in Canada

Postoperative care: Preparing your patient's room

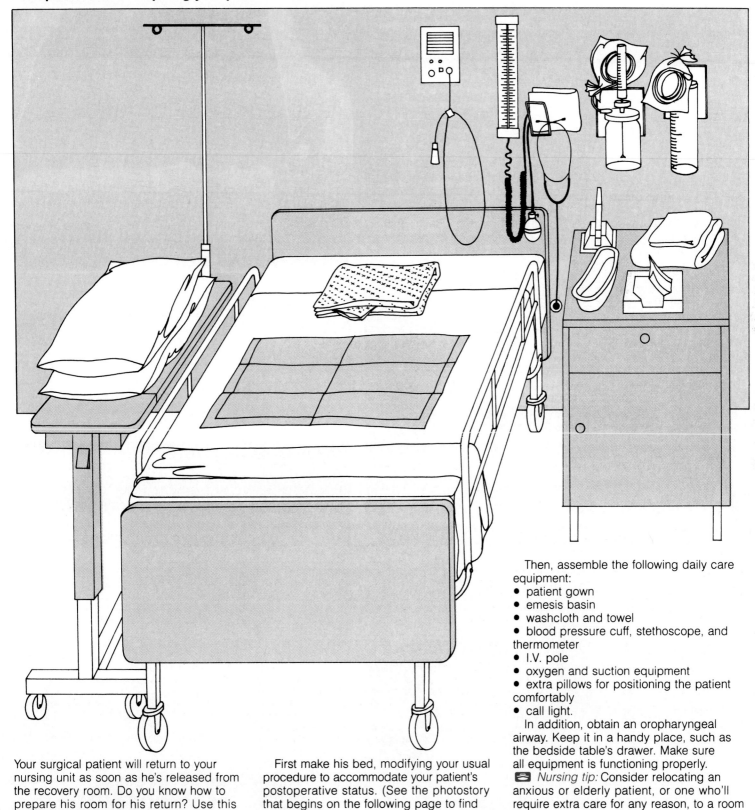

Your surgical patient will return to your nursing unit as soon as he's released from the recovery room. Do you know how to prepare his room for his return? Use this illustration as a guide.

First make his bed, modifying your usual procedure to accommodate your patient's postoperative status. (See the photostory that begins on the following page to find out how.)

Then, assemble the following daily care equipment:
• patient gown
• emesis basin
• washcloth and towel
• blood pressure cuff, stethoscope, and thermometer
• I.V. pole
• oxygen and suction equipment
• extra pillows for positioning the patient comfortably
• call light.

In addition, obtain an oropharyngeal airway. Keep it in a handy place, such as the bedside table's drawer. Make sure all equipment is functioning properly.

Nursing tip: Consider relocating an anxious or elderly patient, or one who'll require extra care for any reason, to a room near the nurses' station.

Immediate care

Postoperative techniques: Making the bed

1 *Of course, making the bed for a patient returning from surgery doesn't differ greatly from making a bed for any other patient. But, certain features that you include in the bed-making will facilitate your handling and care of the postop patient. Read the following photostory to learn new tips.*

Before you begin, consider your patient's specific requirements. Is he thin and debilitated? Or, has he had back or hip surgery? If so, provide extra comfort by obtaining a water mattress to use in place of the usual bed mattress. Or, obtain an alternating pressure mattress, egg crate pad, or flotation pad mattress.

Strip the bed of all used linen; deposit it in a linen hamper. Wash your hands.

Then, obtain the clean linen pictured below: two bedsheets; one or two rubber sheets, depending on expected drainage; two or three drawsheets, depending on expected drainage; bed-saver pads; blanket; pillowcase; and pillow. You may also obtain a bed cradle, to keep the top linens off the patient's legs, and extra pillows and pillowcases for positioning. Set the linen on a clean, dry surface.

Important: Make sure the rubber sheet is unsoiled. If it's not, obtain a clean one.

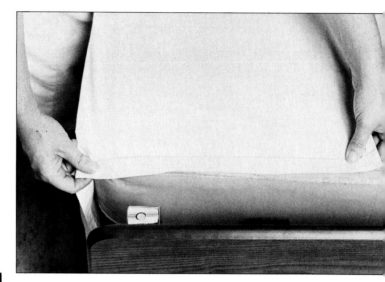

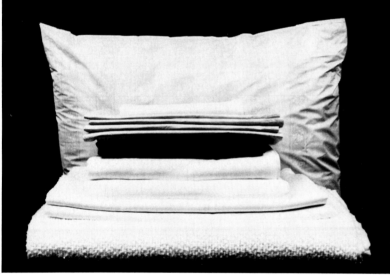

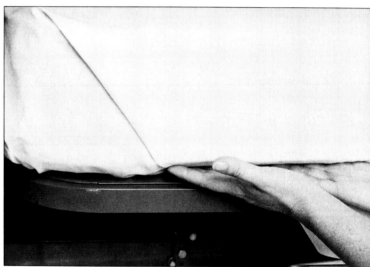

2 Now, standing at the side of the bed, place the bottom sheet over one-half of the mattress, as the nurse is doing here. To help reduce dust-particle activity, make only half of the bed at a time. Never shake the sheet.

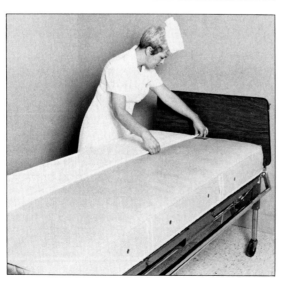

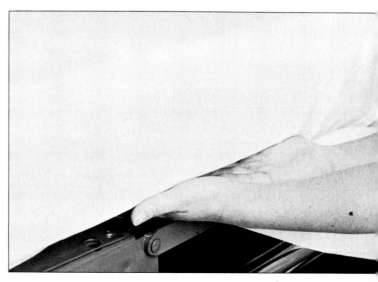

3 Position the bottom edge of the sheet (hemmed edge down) even with the foot of the mattress. Carefully unfold the bottom sheet so the top edge hangs 8" to 10" (20.3 to 25 cm) over the head of the mattress.

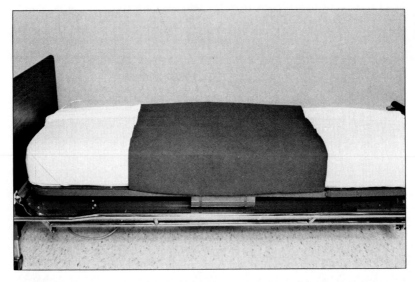

6 Because wound drainage commonly occurs with a postop patient, use a rubber sheet to protect the bottom sheet. Center the rubber sheet midway between the head and foot of the bed.
Note: If the patient's had surgery above his chest, or below his knees, you should place a second rubber sheet in the area of expected drainage.

4 Miter the sheet's top corner. Tuck the sheet's mitered corner under the mattress as far as possible.

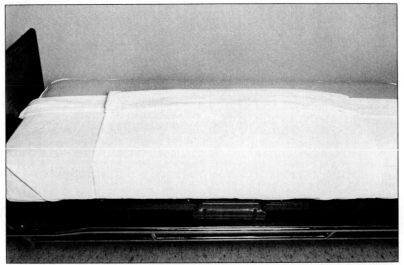

7 Use a drawsheet to protect your patient from the uncomfortable feel of the rubber. Position the drawsheet directly over the rubber sheet, midway between the head and foot of the bed.
Note: If you've used a second rubber sheet, remember to cover it with a second drawsheet.
Unfold the drawsheet toward you. Tightly tuck both the drawsheet's side and the rubber sheet's edge under the mattress.

5 Then, tightly tuck the entire side of the sheet under the mattress, moving from the top mattress corner to the bottom mattress corner.
Note: Does your hospital use fitted bottom sheets? Unfold the fitted sheet across the bed. Fit the four corners of the sheet over the four corners of the mattress. Tightly tuck in both sides of the sheet, working from the head of the bed to the foot.

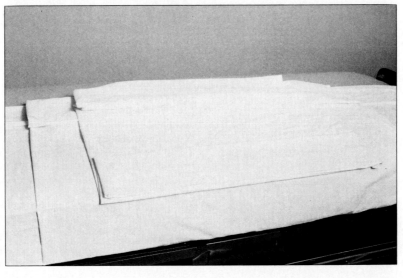

8 Equip the bed with a turning sheet for use in turning and positioning the patient. To do so, fold a drawsheet in half from top to bottom. Position the turning sheet so that its folded edge will rest underneath the patient's shoulders while its bottom edges will rest underneath his hips. Fanfold the side of the turning sheet so it rests on the side of the bed. You can grip the sheet by these fanfolds when you're ready to turn the patient.
Repeat steps 3 through 8 on the other side of the bed.

Immediate care

Postoperative techniques: Making the bed continued

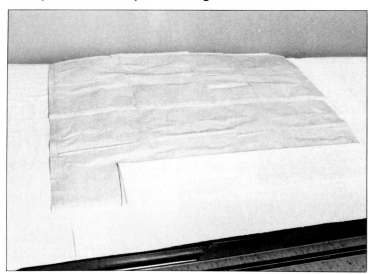

9 Now that the bottom sheets are in place, you may place bed-saver pads over the sheets, in areas of expected drainage.

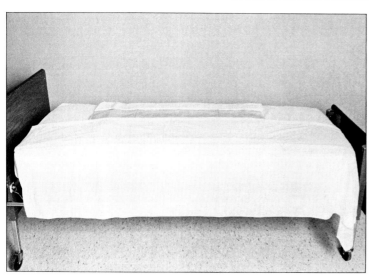

10 Next, arrange the top covers on the bed. Do so by placing the top sheet lengthwise over the drawsheet, so that the upper edge (wide hemmed edge) of the top sheet is flush with the head of the mattress. The bottom of the sheet should extend over the foot of the bed by 8″ to 10″ (20.3 to 25 cm).

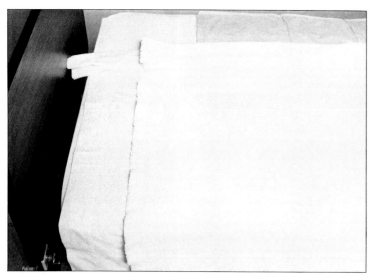

11 Because anesthesia causes vasoconstriction, the postop patient may feel cold. So, use a blanket instead of a bedspread to cover the top sheet. Position the blanket over the top sheet, making sure the blanket's top edge is 5″ to 8″ (12.7 to 20.3 cm) below the sheet's edge.

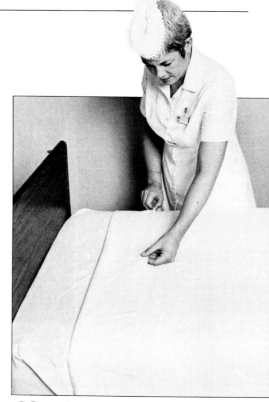

12 Unfold the top sheet (hemmed side up) and the blanket across the whole bed. Fold the top sheet down over the blanket's edge to form a cuff. But don't tuck in the unfolded sheet and blanket at the bed's bottom and sides. Instead, refold the sheet and blanket together, so that they won't interfere with the patient's transfer from stretcher to bed.

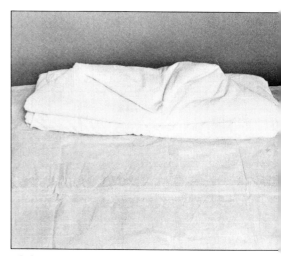

13 Fold these top linens either of two ways. Here's the first way: Fold the top sheet and blanket into thirds by folding down the top third and folding up the bottom third. Bring the side corners to the center of the bed's side, to form a triangle that extends over the bed's edge.
Fold the triangle back, and fanfold the remaining sheet to the far sides of the bed, as shown here.

14 Alternatively, you may fold back the top edge of the sheet and blanket so that they're even with the foot of the bed. Then, fanfold the linens, starting at the top of the bed and continuing to the foot.

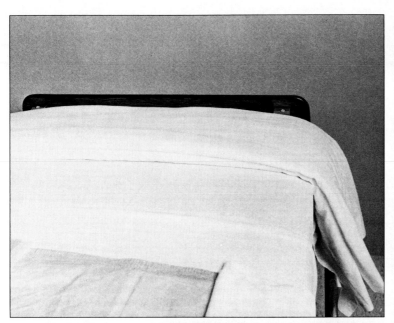

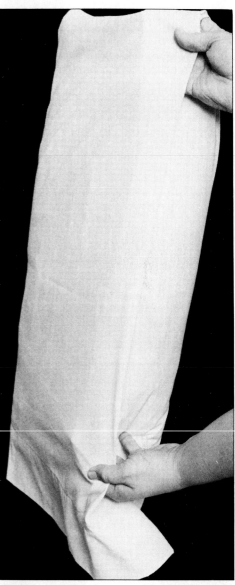

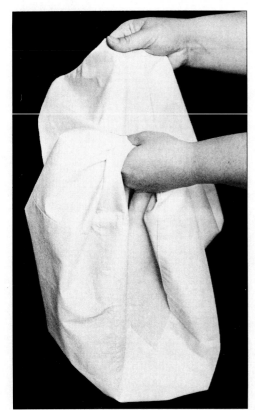

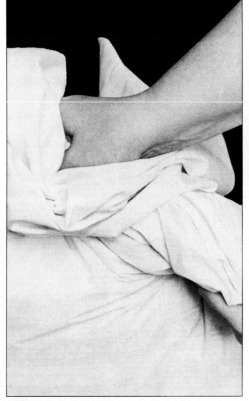

15 Now, you're ready to put the pillow in the pillowcase. To do this, first unfold the pillowcase. Then, with one hand, hold the pillowcase by the bottom seam. Use your other hand to gather the entire length of the pillowcase as the nurse is doing here.

16 Next, using one hand, grasp both the zippered end of the pillow, and the gathered pillowcase (held by the bottom seam). With your other hand, pull the pillowcase over the pillow. Be careful not to let the pillow or case touch your uniform. *Never* hold the pillow under your chin.

17 If necessary, make an envelope fold in the pillowcase's side seam so the case fits tightly.

Then, place the pillow on a clean, dry surface. If you do this, the pillow won't get in the way when you transfer the patient from the stretcher to the bed. After the patient's in bed, place the pillow where it's needed.

Place a drawsheet lengthwise over the whole bed, to protect it from dust until the patient's ready to use it.

Finally, move away from the bedside any obstruction that might interfere with the patient's easy transfer from the stretcher to the bed. Also, position the bed at the angle that will make it most accessible for patient transfer.

Immediate care

Receiving a patient from the recovery room

Suppose you work in a medical/surgical nursing unit, and you're waiting for a patient to return from surgery. When he's ready to leave the recovery room, the recovery room nurse should notify you by telephone. She'll tell you his name; the surgical procedure performed; the type of anesthetic used; his vital signs, level of consciousness, and general condition; whether any I.V. lines, catheters, or drainage tubes are present; and any other pertinent information. This information will permit you to anticipate any special patient needs and obtain appropriate equipment.

When your patient actually arrives in your nursing unit, assist with his transfer from the stretcher to the bed. (See the photostory beginning below.)

As you help with the transfer, begin assessing your patient. For example, note his overall muscle coordination, his general level of consciousness, and his skin color. After he's in bed, complete your assessment,

using the guidelines indicated on pages 60 and 61. Repeat this assessment as often as your hospital policy requires. Usually, you'll assess your patient at least every 15 minutes the first hour, every 30 minutes for the next 2 hours, once an hour for 4 hours, and then every 4 hours.

Note: When you compare your patient's vital signs with his previous values, keep in mind that minor variations sometimes occur after transport. For example, he may have an increase in blood pressure, pulse rate, and respiratory rate. However, report any significant changes to the doctor immmediately.

While performing your assessment, be sure to assess your patient for pain, nausea, or vomiting, ability to assume a comfortable position, and sensations of coldness or warmth. Take any steps necessary to decrease the discomfort he's feeling; for example, by providing medication or blankets. (For specific pain relief measures,

see the section beginning on page 70.) Encourage your patient to cough and deep breathe frequently, as you taught him preoperatively.

Keep in mind that the early postoperative period is the most critical phase of the patient's convalescence. During this phase, appearances can be deceptive. Although your patient seems to be sleeping peacefully, he could actually be going into shock. So, don't be lulled into neglecting regular assessments. And, if your patient shows any signs or symptoms of a postoperative complication (no matter how subtle), increase the frequency of your assessments. Document all assessment findings in your nurses' notes.

Before leaving your patient, help ensure his safety by lowering the bed to its lowest position, raising the side rails, and placing a call bell within his reach. Then, notify family members of your patient's return from surgery and his general condition.

Transferring your patient from stretcher to bed

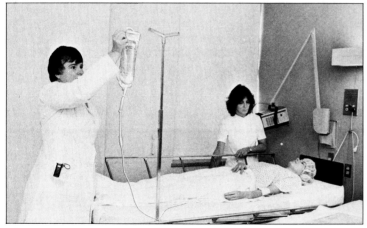

1 *Your patient, Clara Rawlings, who's just had an abdominal hysterectomy, is returning to your unit from the recovery room. Begin your patient care by assisting with her transfer from the stretcher to the bed.*

First, explain the procedure to your patient. Make sure she's lying supine, with her body well-aligned. Then, position the stretcher at one side of the bed. Adjust the bed to stretcher level. Lower the side rail on the side of the stretcher nearest the bed.

Now, check any equipment, such as an indwelling (Foley) catheter or I.V. tubing, to make sure it's not entangled in the bed frame or side rails. Move the I.V. container from the stretcher I.V. pole to the bed frame I.V. pole, as the nurse is doing here. Then, remove the I.V. pole from the stretcher. Have a co-worker position herself near the head of the stretcher. Instruct her to lower the side rail on her side of the stretcher, as she's doing here.

Then, roll the stretcher close to the bed and lock both the bed wheels and the stretcher wheels.

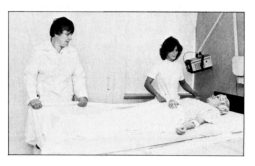

2 Next, loosen the stretcher sheet so it's free of the stretcher. Begin rolling the stretcher sheet toward the patient's side.

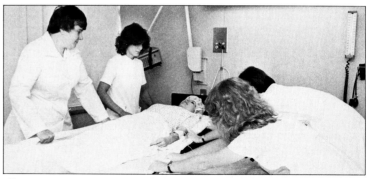

3 Ask two co-workers to stand on the far side of the bed, facing you, and instruct them to roll their side of the stretcher sheet close to the patient's body.

Then, have the co-worker next to you grasp the sheet with her left hand near the patient's ear and her right hand near the patient's abdomen. You should grasp the sheet with your left hand near the patient's hip and your right hand near the patient's calf. This technique evenly distributes the patient's weight between you, and gives the patient added support for her back and abdomen.

4 An alternative method of grasping the sheet, the crossed-arm technique, is illustrated here.

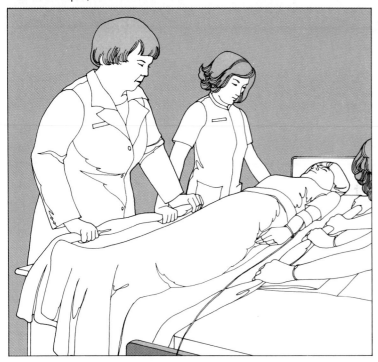

6 On another predetermined signal, lift your patient toward the center of the bed. Carefully lower her into the bed, keeping her body aligned. *Note:* You may need to lift a heavy patient in three stages before you reach the center of the bed.

On another predetermined signal, lift your patient toward the center of the bed. Carefully lower her into the bed, keeping her body aligned. *Note:* You may need to lift a heavy patient in three stages before you reach the center of the bed.

When she's safely positioned in the bed, move the stretcher out of the way. Then, position the patient squarely in the center of the bed, as shown here. Have your co-workers on the opposite side raise the bed's side rail.

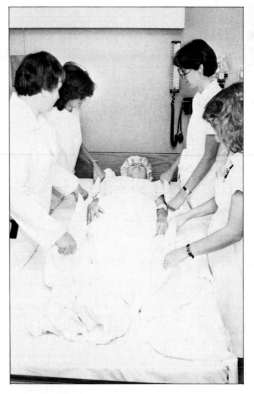

5 Instruct the patient to keep her arms at her side throughout the transfer. Also, tell her to deep breathe during the transfer, to help her relax.

Ask your co-workers on the opposite side of the bed to grasp the sheet in the same way as you and your partner are doing. Make sure you and all co-workers have your feet positioned 2 to 3 feet (60 to 90 cm) apart, and your knees bent.

All ready? On a predetermined signal, slightly lift the patient and move her to the edge of the stretcher. Then, gently lower the patient to the edge of the bed, as shown here.

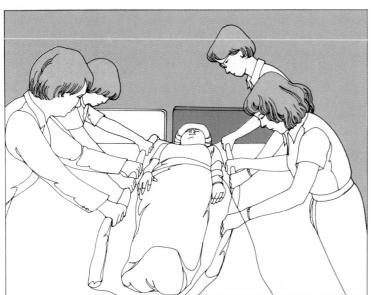

7 Complete the procedure by having your patient turn on her side, using the technique we describe on page 82. Then, roll up the stretcher sheet tightly against her back, as the nurse is doing here. Remove the stretcher sheet from the bed.

Then, position your patient comfortably in the center of the bed. Adjust her top linens and pillow. Perform a thorough postoperative assessment. Raise the side rail on your side of the bed, and place a call bell within her reach.

Finally, document the procedure and your assessment in your nurses' notes.

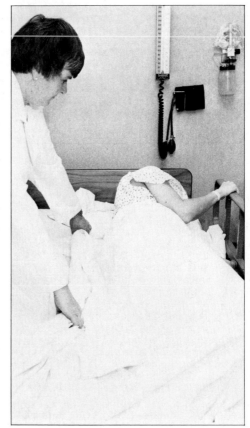

Pain management

The surgical patient almost always feels some postoperative pain. But your pain management can make the crucial difference between extreme suffering and minor discomfort.

Of course, successful pain management depends on your accurate assessment. So, in the box below, we outline a procedure for evaluating your patient's pain.

Then, we'll discuss the general types of analgesics. We'll also give you guidelines for analgesic use, as well as a step-by-step method for administering pain medication. For easy reference, we've provided a chart of commonly-used analgesic drugs.

Do you realize that noninvasive pain-control techniques include old-fashioned comfort measures, as well as more sophisticated distraction and relaxation techniques? In the following pages, we'll tell you how to effectively employ a variety of these techniques.

Finally, you may have heard about alternative pain control technologies. The new EPC®/Dual Electronic Pain Control device provides a substitute for medication. We'll describe the equipment for you and then show you how to use it.

MINI-ASSESSMENT

Assessing your patient's pain

Your patient's just returned from the recovery room. As the general anesthetic's effects continue to wear off, he begins to wince with pain. You're not surprised. Most postoperative patients experience some degree of pain, because of surgery's invasive nature.

Of course, you want to do your best to provide pain relief. As your first step, assess your patient's pain carefully. Then, you'll know better how to alleviate it. The following guidelines will aid in your assessment.
• First, consider the type of surgery the patient's had. Different types of surgery cause different kinds of pain. After abdominal surgery, incisional pain may be more severe on the first and second postoperative day, whereas deeper visceral pain (pain affecting internal organs) and gas pains are more severe on the third and fourth days. If you keep such a pattern in mind, the patient's statements about pain will be clearer to you. But, don't let your preconceptions affect your assessment. Remember to listen to your patient's statements. After all, he's the one experiencing the pain. Also, keep in mind any information supplied by your preoperative assessment and your assessment of how he tolerates pain.
• Observe your patient for any physical or psychological signs that may indicate pain. Does he seem restless and irritable? Is he picking at his covers? Is he wincing, grimacing, or stiffening his body? Is he groaning, moaning, or crying? Has his heart rate or blood pressure increased since your last assessment? Has his respiratory rate increased? Are his pupils dilated? Has his skin color or skin temperature changed? Remember, a patient in pain may show pallor and diaphoresis.
• When your patient's alert enough to respond, ask him to describe the quality of the pain. Is it a throbbing or stabbing pain, a dull ache, or a cramping spasm?
• Ask him to describe the pain's location. Have him point to the affected area of his body, if he can. Or, if he's having difficulty localizing the pain, have him indicate which areas are pain-free. He'll probably be able to isolate superficial or bone pain more easily than visceral or somatic pain.
• How intense is the pain? It could range anywhere from mild to unbearable.
• Can the patient describe any other feelings associated with the pain?
• Does a change of position or any other comfort measure diminish his pain?
• After the patient's received his medication, you'll need to determine how it affects his pain. Is the patient experiencing adequate relief? If so, for how long? Does the patient display any adverse effects? Assess him every 30 to 45 minutes after administering pain medication. The doctor will rely heavily on your assessment in deciding whether to adjust the dosage or change to another drug.

Learning about analgesics

As you know, analgesic medication is used to provide pain relief without loss of consciousness. Your postoperative patient will probably need analgesics to see him through the first several days of pain. For detailed information about commonly-used analgesics, refer to the chart beginning on page 73.

In prescribing the appropriate analgesic, the doctor can choose between two basic types: narcotics and nonnarcotics. How do they differ? First of all, nonnarcotics act primarily on the patient's peripheral nervous system, although they have some effect on his central nervous system (CNS). (In the illustration on the next page, pain pathways from peripheral areas are shown in black.) Nonnarcotics provide a relatively small measure of pain relief. But they work well for mild to moderate pain. And they cause no major CNS side effects, such as sedation, respiratory depression, or physiologic dependency. However, aspirin (A.S.A.), a commonly-used nonnarcotic, may cause local symptoms such as stomach irritation and bleeding.

Nonnarcotics, including acetaminophen (Tylenol*), also act as antipyretics, which can be an advantage or a disadvantage. They'll help reduce a high fever, but they may also, by suppressing fever, mask the first signs of infection. Aspirin also has anti-inflammatory properties which makes it particularly effective against arthritic pain. You'll almost always give nonnarcotics orally, although you may occasionally give them rectally.

Narcotics act primarily on the central nervous system. (See the pain pathways shown in blue in the illustration on the next page.) The doctor prescribes them for severe pain that nonnarcotics can't greatly affect. However, narcotics can cause major CNS side effects, including nausea and vomiting, constipation, sedation, respiratory depression, and physiologic dependency and tolerance. Side effects increase, of course, if the patient inadvertently receives a dose beyond his individual tolerance, or if he has an allergy to a particular drug. What's the correct dosage? It varies greatly, depending on the narcotic's potency, and how efficiently the patient's system metabolizes the narcotic. The initial dose may need to be adjusted.

You'll usually give narcotics by injection, either subcutaneously or intramuscularly, rather than orally, for faster pain relief. But, under certain circumstances (for example, if the patient's a hemophiliac, or if he's a child) the doctor may find the oral route preferable. Rarely, he may also order narcotics I.V., to provide immediate relief of intense pain.

Since narcotics and nonnarcotics act on different components of the patient's nervous system, their combined effect is synergistic. In other words, when the medications are combined, they have a better pain-relieving effect than they would if they weren't combined.

If a patient has severe pain and can take medication orally, the doctor might order a nonnarcotic to supplement a narcotic injection. This way, the patient can receive a smaller dose of narcotic medication, which reduces the risk of side effects. If a patient has mild pain that becomes severe, the doctor might replace a nonnarcotic with a narcotic.

**Narcotic agonists
and narcotic agonist-antagonists**
Narcotics can be subdivided into two groups: agonists and agonist-antagonists. An agonist is a drug that functions solely as a narcotic, acting on the central nervous system to relieve pain as we've already explained. Morphine sulfate* is an example of a narcotic agonist.

But, a new type of narcotic has recently been developed. This is the agonist-antagonist. On page 75, we've presented an example: butorphanol tartrate (Stadol). This drug functions as an agonist when given alone. But, when combined with a standard narcotic agonist, such as morphine sulfate, the drug acts as an antagonist, counteracting the morphine sulfate's effects. This means that if your patient developed a physiologic dependency on an agonist, and his doctor ordered an agonist-antagonist, you would administer the second drug only with extreme caution. If butorphanol tartrate were substituted for morphine sulfate too quickly, your patient might experience both withdrawal symptoms and inadequate pain relief. How severely he'd react would reflect the degree of his drug dependency and the strength of the butorphanol tartrate's antagonist action.

To protect your patient from any ill effects, check his recent medication history *before* you start giving him agonist-antagonists. Find out which narcotic he's been taking. For a clue about his physiologic dependency, check the length of time he's been taking the narcotic. Note also whether his dose has gradually increased, or whether the interval between injections has gradually decreased.

Also, when you give an agonist-antagonist to a patient, even if he hasn't been taking any narcotics, be prepared for negative psychic reactions such as hallucinations. Narcotic agonist-antagonists can also cause all the side effects of a narcotic agonist, including respiratory depression.

Note: If your patient does experience respiratory depression from either type of narcotic, give him naloxone (Narcan*), as ordered. Naloxone counteracts both agonists and agonist-antagonists.

Midbrain

Lower medulla

Cervical cord

Pain management

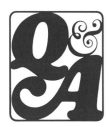

Using analgesics effectively

Do you feel uncertain about giving pain medication? For example, are you sure that your patient's receiving just the right amount? When giving a narcotic medication, do you worry about addiction? If the doctor orders a medication to be administered rectally, do you know why? The following dialogue may answer some of your questions.

Q: When my patient first complains of pain, should I give him medication promptly, or hold off until the pain's really severe?
A: The key to effective pain management is prevention. Give your patient adequate medication before the pain becomes severe, because the worse he feels, the more medication he'll probably require to relieve his pain. More medication means more drug-associated side effects.

Q: What constitutes adequate medication?
A: You're giving adequate medication when you provide your patient continuous relief from severe pain, without serious side effects. The correct drug and dosage, of course, depend on the patient. As you know, pain tolerance varies from patient to patient. In addition, each patient's system metabolizes drugs differently. An older patient's system will metabolize a drug more slowly than an adolescent's system; as a result, an older patient may receive fewer immediate benefits and greater long-lasting ones. Or, a patient's system might not successfully metabolize a certain drug; for example, oxycodone hydrochloride (Percodan*), so he'll require a different drug altogether.

Q: How can I help ensure the appropriate dosage for my patient?
A: After you've given a prescribed dose, assess your patient as instructed here and on page 70.
Ask yourself: Does my patient feel immediate relief, but begin to feel pain within an hour? Check whether the order permits you to increase the dose. If not, ask the doctor to write a new order, either increasing the dose limits or decreasing the interval between injections. Suppose your patient says his pain has decreased dramatically, but he seems very groggy. Decrease the dosage, if permitted, or do so after obtaining the order from the doctor.
If your patient experiences *no* pain relief, *increase* the dosage if the order permits, or do so after obtaining the order from the doctor. If an increased dosage still provides no pain relief for your patient, the doctor will probably order a different medication.

Q: Suppose the patient continually gets a large enough dosage so that he never has severe pain. Will he become addicted to the drug?
A: Probably not. Addiction happens rarely among long-term pain medication users; only about 1% of them become addicted. And, a patient who's had elective surgery will usually receive narcotics for only a few days, provided he doesn't have complications. He'll probably stop taking the medication without feeling much effect. However, the patient who takes medication for 10 to 14 days may develop a physiologic dependency and tolerance for the drug. But, although these physiologic adaptations are components of the addictive pattern, addiction also involves a very great psychological dependency, which few patients develop. For most patients, withdrawal symptoms disappear within a few days. Tolerance decreases to a normal level within a few weeks.

Q: What about administering analgesic medication rectally?
A: You may administer analgesic medication rectally, in the form of a rectal suppository. You might use this route for a patient who's just undergone abdominal surgery, or to administer nonnarcotics for mild discomfort or fever. But, you'll rarely give *narcotic* medications rectally, because drug absorption varies greatly and may be incomplete. The narcotic medication most commonly given rectally is oxymorphone hydrochloride (Numorphan). Try to give any rectal medication immediately after a bowel movement, to ensure rapid absorption of the drug.

*Available in both the United States and in Canada

How to administer analgesics

Administering analgesics? Use this step-by-step guide. For information on specific drugs, read the following chart.
• First, assess your patient to determine the location, intensity, and quality of pain (for example, sharp, dull, throbbing, or stabbing). Note any associated signs and symptoms, such as a change in vital signs. Be alert for any nonverbal cues that might indicate pain, such as restlessness, irritability, or grimacing.
• Familiarize yourself with prescribed medication. Review its properties. Note especially its speed of onset, peak of action, duration of action, and adverse effects. Check the patient's medical history to try to anticipate the drug's effect on the patient. Allergies, alcoholism, or drug abuse, as well as ability to tolerate stress, are relevant factors. Verify that the dosage is within the safe and effective range, considering the patient's weight and his age.
• Check the patient's record to see when medication was last administered. Determine the time elapsed since the last dose and give the medication according to the prescribed intervals. Usually, 3 to 4 hours must elapse between doses, even when the doctor specifies that you give the medication as needed.
• Review the patient's care plan to see if the injection fits conveniently into his schedule of activities. For example, the patient will appreciate receiving an injection timed to relieve the additional pain associated with ambulation, deep breathing and coughing exercises, or dressing changes.
• Prepare the drug as ordered, depending on administration route. Check for the 5 Rs: right patient, right drug, right dose, right route, and right time.
• Administer the drug, as ordered.
• Then, on the patient's medication record, note the drug's name, the dose you've given, the time you gave it, and your initials. Also, sign your name at the appropriate place on the medication record.
• To evaluate the analgesic's effectiveness, assess the patient within 30 minutes. Check him for adverse effects, such as nausea and vomiting, urticaria, rashes, respiratory depression, or oversedation. Document your observations in your nurses' notes.
• Subsequently, reassess the patient's pain at 30- to 45-minute intervals. Note the peak and duration of the drug's action.
Note: Since an elderly or debilitated patient's system metabolizes drugs slowly, you can expect delayed drug action and delayed adverse effects. Elderly patients also seem to have a greater sensitivity to analgesics than other adults. They usually require reduced dosages.
• Notify the doctor if the patient's pain remains unrelieved, or if he has an allergic reaction to the medication.

Nurses' guide to analgesic drugs

Aspirin
(A.S.A., Ecotrin*, Empirin)

Classification
Nonnarcotic

Indications and dosage
For mild pain
Adults: 325 to 650 mg P.O. or rectally every 4 hours, as needed.

Side effects
Prolonged bleeding time; occult bleeding; nausea, vomiting, and gastrointestinal (GI) distress; diaphoresis; abnormal liver function; rash; hypersensitivity manifested by anaphylaxis; tinnitus and hearing loss (first signs of toxicosis)

Interactions
• With ammonium chloride (and other urine acidifiers), blood levels of aspirin-metabolic products increase. Monitor patient for aspirin toxicosis.
• With antacids (and other urine alkalinizers), blood levels of aspirin-metabolic products decrease. Monitor patient for decreased aspirin effect.
• With anticoagulants, hemorrhage risk increases. Avoid using together, if possible.
• With a narcotic, it enhances the narcotic's pain-relieving effect.

Precautions
• Contraindicated in GI ulcer, GI bleeding, aspirin hypersensitivity.
• Use cautiously in patients with hypoprothrombinemia, vitamin K deficiency, blood dyscrasia, asthma with nasal polyps (may cause severe bronchospasm), and Hodgkin's disease (may cause profound hypothermia).

Nursing considerations
• Give with food, milk, antacid, or large glass of water to reduce GI side effects.
• Don't give with an alcoholic elixir; alcohol may increase GI bleeding.
• Because enteric-coated aspirin (Ecotrin*), or timed-release preparations are absorbed erratically, they are not appropriate for long-term therapy.
• May mask fever because it's antipyretic.
• Helps relieve pain caused by inflammation.

Acetaminophen
(Tylenol*)

Classification
Nonnarcotic

Indications and dosage
For mild pain
Adults: 325 to 600 mg every 4 hours, as needed, up to a maximum dosage of 2.6 g daily.

Side effects
Rash; urticaria; severe liver toxicosis (with massive doses)

Interactions
• With a narcotic, it enhances the narcotic's pain-relieving effect.

Precautions
• High doses or unsupervised chronic use can cause liver damage. Excessive ingestion of alcoholic beverages may enhance liver toxicosis.

Nursing considerations
• May mask fever because it's antipyretic. But, unlike aspirin, acetaminophen has no anti-inflammatory effect.
• Warn patient that high doses or unsupervised long-term use can cause liver damage.
• Warn patient that excessive ingestion of alcoholic beverages with drug may damage his liver.

Zomepirac sodium
(Zomax)

Classification
Nonnarcotic

Indications and dosage
For mild to moderately severe pain
Adults: 100 mg P.O. every 4 to 6 hours as needed, up to a maximum of 600 mg per day. (For mild pain, 50 mg every 4 to 6 hours may be sufficient.)

Side effects
Tinnitus; taste change; drowsiness; dizziness; insomnia; paresthesia; nervousness; edema; hypertension; cardiac irregularity; palpitations; nausea; vomiting; diarrhea; dyspepsia; constipation; flatulence; anorexia; urinary frequency; elevated blood urea nitrogen (BUN) and creatinine levels; urinary tract infection; vaginitis; rash; pruritus; chills

Interactions
• Aspirin may decrease zomepirac sodium's efficacy.

Precautions
• Contraindicated for patients in whom aspirin and other nonsteroidal anti-inflammatory drugs induce bronchospasm, rhinitis, urticaria, or other sensitivity reactions.
• Use cautiously in patients with a history of GI bleeding, fluid retention, hypertension, and heart failure.

Nursing considerations
• Although this drug is a nonnarcotic analgesic, it has narcotic potency. According to several studies, it's as effective as morphine.
• Does not appear to be addictive.
• May mask fever because it's antipyretic.
• May reduce pain caused by inflammation.
• If GI signs and symptoms occur, give subsequent doses with food or antacids.

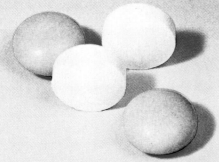
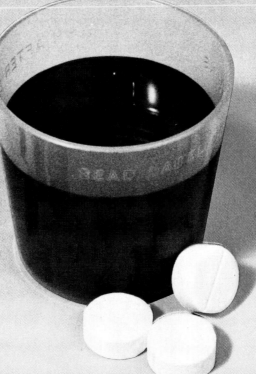
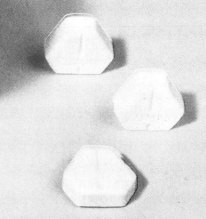

*Available in both the United States and in Canada

Pain management

Nurses' guide to analgesic drugs continued

Oxycodone hydrochloride
(Available in U.S. only in combination with aspirin as Percodan*, and with acetaminophen as Percocet-5, Tylox.)

Classification
Narcotic (agonist)

Indications and dosage
For moderate pain
Adults: 1 to 2 tablets P.O every 6 hours, as needed.

Side effects
Sedation; clouded sensorium; euphoria; respiratory depression; physical dependence; convulsions (with large doses); hypotension; bradycardia; nausea or vomiting; constipation; paralytic ileus; urinary retention

Interactions
• When used with anticoagulants, oxycodone hydrochloride products containing aspirin (Percodan*) may increase anticoagulant effect. Use together cautiously, and monitor patient's blood-clotting times.
• Central nervous system (CNS) depression is increased when drug is used with general anesthetics, other narcotic analgesics, tranquilizers, sedatives, hypnotics, tricyclic antidepressants, MAO inhibitors, or alcohol. When combining oxycodone hydrochloride with these drugs, reduce oxycodone hydrochloride dose. Use together only with extreme caution and closely monitor patient's response.

Precautions
• Use with extreme caution in patients with head injury, increased intracranial pressure, seizures, asthma, chronic obstructive pulmonary disease (COPD), alcoholism, prostatic hypertrophy, severe hepatic or renal disease, acute abdominal conditions, urethral stricture, hypothyroidism, Addison's disease, cardiac arrhythmias, reduced blood volume, or toxic psychosis. Also, use with caution in elderly or debilitated patients.

Nursing considerations
• Provides high level of analgesia when given P.O., but also carries high risk of addiction.
• For full analgesic effect, give before patient has severe pain.
• Give after meals or with milk.
• Monitor circulatory and respiratory status and bowel function. Don't give if patient's respiratory rate is less than 10 breaths per minute.
• Warn ambulatory patients to avoid activities that require alertness.

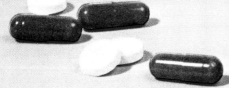

Codeine phosphate, codeine sulfate

Classification
Narcotic (agonist)

Indications and dosage
For mild to moderate pain
Adults: 15 to 60 mg P.O. every 4 hours, as needed. 15 to 60 mg codeine phosphate subcutaneously or I.M. every 4 hours, as needed.

Side effects
Sedation; clouded sensorium; euphoria; respiratory depression; physical dependence; convulsions (with large doses); hypotension; bradycardia; nausea or vomiting; constipation; paralytic ileus; urinary retention

Interactions
• CNS depression increases when drug is used with general anesthetics, other narcotic analgesics, tranquilizers, sedatives, hypnotics, alcohol, tricyclic antidepressants, or MAO inhibitors. Use together with extreme caution, and closely monitor patient's response.
• With aspirin and acetominophen, pain-relieving effects are enhanced.

Precautions
• Use with extreme caution in patients with head injuries, increased intracranial pressure, hepatic or renal disease, hypothyroidism, Addison's disease, acute alcoholism, seizures, severe CNS depression, bronchial asthma, COPD, respiratory depression, or shock. Also, use cautiously in elderly or debilitated patients.

Nursing considerations
• Don't administer discolored injection solution.
• Monitor respiratory and circulatory status, as well as urine output and bowel function.
• Warn ambulatory patients to avoid activities that require alertness.

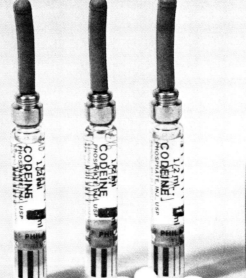

Morphine sulfate

Classification
Narcotic (agonist)

Indications and dosage
For severe pain
Adults: 5 to 15 mg I.M. or subcutaneously every 4 hours, as needed.
I.V.: 5 to 15 mg diluted in 4 to 5 ml water, injected slowly over 4 to 5 minutes. Give every 4 hours, as needed.
P.O.: 30 to 60 mg every 4 hours, as needed.

Side effects
Sedation; clouded sensorium; euphoria; convulsions (with large doses); respiratory depression; physical dependence; hypotension; bradycardia; nausea; vomiting; constipation; paralytic ileus; urinary retention

Interactions
• Drug may cause respiratory depression, hypotension, or profound sedation when used with general anesthetics, tranquilizers, sedatives, hypnotics, alcohol, tricyclic antidepressants, or MAO inhibitors. Use together only with extreme caution. When combining morphine sulfate with any of these drugs, reduce morphine sulfate dose and closely monitor patient's response.

Precautions
• Use with extreme caution in patients with head injury, increased intracranial pressure, seizures, asthma, COPD, alcoholism, prostatic hypertrophy, severe hepatic or renal disease, acute abdominal conditions, hypothyroidism, Addison's disease, urethral stricture, cardiac arrhythmias, reduced blood volume, or toxic psychosis. Also, use cautiously in elderly or debilitated patients.

Nursing considerations
• Have narcotic antagonist naloxone (Narcan*) and resuscitative equipment available, in case respiratory depression occurs.
• Monitor circulatory and respiratory status and bowel functions. Don't give drug if respiratory rate is less than 10 breaths per minute.
• Warn ambulatory patients to avoid activities that require alertness.
• Drug of choice in relieving pain from myocardial infarction. May cause transient decrease in blood pressure.
Important: Giving narcotics I.V. may be the doctor's responsibility. Check hospital policy.

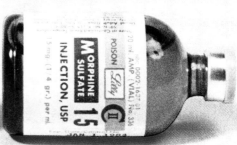

*Available in both the United States and in Canada

Meperidine hydrochloride
(Demerol*)

Classification
Narcotic (agonist)

Indications and dosage
For moderate to severe pain
Adults: 50 to 150 mg P.O., I.M., or subcutaneously every 3 to 4 hours, as needed.

Side effects
Sedation; clouded sensorium; euphoria; convulsions (with large doses); respiratory depression; physical dependence; hypotension; bradycardia; nausea; vomiting; constipation; paralytic ileus; urinary retention; pain at injection site; local tissue irritation and induration after subcutaneous injection; phlebitis after I.V. injection

Interactions
• With MAO inhibitors and isoniazid (INH), severe or fatal CNS excitation or depression may occur. Don't use these drugs together.
• Drug may cause respiratory depression, hypotension, profound sedation, or coma when used with other narcotic analgesics, general anesthetics, phenothiazines, sedatives, hypnotics, tricyclic antidepressants, and alcohol. Use together only with extreme caution, and closely monitor patient's response. When using meperidine hydrochloride (Demerol*) with any of these drugs, reduce meperidine hydrochloride dose.

Precautions
• Contraindicated if patient has used MAO inhibitors within 14 days.
• Use with extreme caution in patients with increased intracranial pressure, shock, CNS depression, head injury, asthma, COPD, respiratory depression, supraventricular tachycardia, seizure, acute abdominal condition, hepatic or renal disease, hypothyroidism, Addison's disease, urethral stricture, prostatic hypertrophy, or alcoholism. Also, use cautiously in elderly or debilitated patients and children under age 12.

Nursing considerations
• Physically incompatible with barbiturates. Don't mix together in same syringe.
• Oral dose is less than half as effective as parenteral dose. Doctor will order I.M. dose, if possible. When changing from parenteral route to oral route, dose should be increased.
• Doctor may (rarely) order meperidine hydrochloride given slow I.V. for severe pain. Administer as a diluted solution.
• Syrup has local anesthetic effect. To prevent numbing, give with a full glass of water.
• Monitor respiratory and cardiovascular status carefully. Don't give if patient's respirations are less than 10 breaths per minute.
• Keep naloxone (Narcan*) narcotic antagonist available when giving drug I.V.
• Warn ambulatory patients to avoid activities that require alertness.

Nursing considerations (continued)
• Meperidine hydrochloride and active metabolite normeperidine accumulate in patients with renal failure. Monitor these patients for possible increased toxic effect.
• Watch for withdrawal symptoms if administration is stopped abruptly after long-term use.
• May be administered in combination with promethazine hydrochloride (Phenergan*) as Mepergan. Promethazine hydrochloride potentiates meperidine hydrochloride's analgesic effects, and may prevent nausea and vomiting, which are common side effects of meperidine hydrochloride.
Important: Giving narcotics I.V. may be the doctor's responsibility. Check your hospital's policy before administering narcotics by this route.

Butorphanol tartrate
(Stadol)

Classification
Nonnarcotic (agonist-antagonist)

Indications and dosage
Moderate to severe pain
Adults: I.M.: 1 to 4 mg every 3 to 4 hours, as needed.
I.V.: 0.5 to 2 mg every 3 to 4 hours, as needed.

Side effects
Sedation; respiratory depression; headache; vertigo; floating sensation; lethargy; confusion; nervousness; bizarre dreams; agitation; euphoria; hallucinations; flushing; palpitations; diplopia; blurred vision; nausea; vomiting; dry mouth; rash; hives; diaphoresis; clammy skin

Interactions
• With narcotics, has an antagonist effect. Do not give to a patient being treated with narcotics.

Precautions
• Contraindicated in narcotic addiction; may precipitate narcotic abstinence syndrome.
• Use cautiously in patients with head injury, increased intracranial pressure, acute myocardial infarction, ventricular dysfunction, coronary insufficiency, respiratory disease, respiratory depression, and renal or hepatic dysfunction.

Nursing considerations
• Subcutaneous route not recommended.
• Respiratory depression does not increase with increased dosage.
• Drug dependency unlikely to occur.
• Also approved for use as a preoperative medication and as the analgesic component of balanced anesthetics.

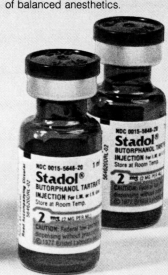

Pain management

Learning about noninvasive pain-control techniques

You may feel that nothing but a narcotic injection will *really* relieve your patient's pain. If so, you're disregarding the brain's ability to produce its own narcotic-like substances called endorphins.

Like narcotics, endorphins form chemical attachments to chemoreceptor sites in the brain and spinal cord. These sites are abundant in the limbic areas of the brain, which regulate emotions, as well as in cognitive areas of the brain. (See the illustration at right for some areas where chemoreceptors can be found.)

So like narcotics, endorphins probably relieve pain by altering the patient's perception of pain, as well as his emotional response to it. Many simple noninvasive techniques can help stimulate endorphin release in your patient, thereby reducing his pain.

Implement one or more of these pain-relieving techniques to prevent or treat your patient's pain. If your patient still requires medication, continue the noninvasive measures. Using them may de-

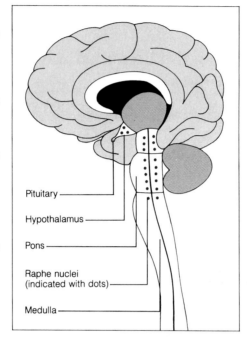

Pituitary

Hypothalamus

Pons

Raphe nuclei
(indicated with dots)

Medulla

crease the medication required.

Of course, you should never deny a patient any medication he needs. But, by using noninvasive techniques, you can reduce or avoid the side effects associated with medication.

What are the specific measures you can use against pain? You've already employed one psychological technique—preoperative teaching. Adequately instructing your patient about his surgery goes a long way toward reducing his anxiety, which should alleviate some of his pain.

Other effective pain-relieving techniques include such comfort measures as positioning, back rubs, creating a comfortable environment in the patient's room, and spending time with the patient. Never neglect these measures. But, if they prove insufficient, teach your patient more systematic techniques for distraction or relaxation, or provide cutaneous stimulation. Read the following information for details.

Using comfort measures to control pain

When caring for your postoperative patient, take time to perform the measures described here. They'll promote his well-being and speed his recovery.

You may feel that these tasks consume too much valuable time. But comfort measures need not be time-consuming if every staff member helps. Remember, all your nursing care rests on the foundation of patient comfort.
- First, position the patient for greatest comfort. In doing so, consider how he was positioned for surgery. If he was uncomfortably positioned for an extended period, find an alternative position that won't stretch or strain the same muscles or aggravate the same pressure points. Usually, you'll assist the patient to a back or side-lying position, whichever he prefers. If you turn him on his side, use a pillow to support him in front and back. Elevate the head of his bed, and support his head with pillows. Use additional pillows to elevate any affected extremities. *Important:* Never place pillows under the patient's knees, or raise the bed under the patient's knees, in any way that might restrict circulation. This increases the risk of thrombophlebitis.
- If your patient's capable, encourage him to frequently turn himself in bed. If he can't, tell him to call for help. Or, consider installing an overhead trapeze, so he can easily change position by himself.
- Create a comfortable, quiet environment in the patient's room. To do this, close the window shades if the patient seems bothered by bright light. Check the room temperature periodically and adjust the thermostat if the room's too hot or cold for the patient. Reduce the radio or television volume. Obtain the

patient's and his family's cooperation in limiting the number of visitors and the length of their stay.
- Attend to the patient's personal care. Surprisingly, simple actions such as applying a cool cloth to the patient's head, smoothing out his bed to reduce uncomfortable wrinkles, and giving mouth care can reduce your patient's pain. All these measures combined help reduce discomfort perceptions that aggravate his pain.
- Give the patient a back rub, if he finds back rubs relaxing. But, first explain the procedure to him. Then, position him so he's lying on his stomach or side. Or, if these positions are contraindicated, lean the patient forward in bed. Apply lotion or powder to your hands to decrease friction and increase the back rub's effectiveness. Using the palms of both hands, begin the back rub at his sacrum and work up to his shoulders. Massage gently, with a circular motion. Pay particular attention to prominent pressure points such as his scapulae, sacrum, and iliac crests. Continue the back massage for about 5 minutes, unless the patient asks you to stop.
- Spend time with the patient, even when you're not specifically giving care. The presence of another person provides both reassurance and distraction, which can alter the patient's pain perception. When you visit the patient, express your interest in him and in the way he's feeling. Use touch (by holding your patient's hand, for example) to communicate that you care. If he doesn't feel like talking, merely sit quietly with him. But don't ignore him, or give him the impression that you're preoccupied. Always be ready to respond if he needs to be comforted.

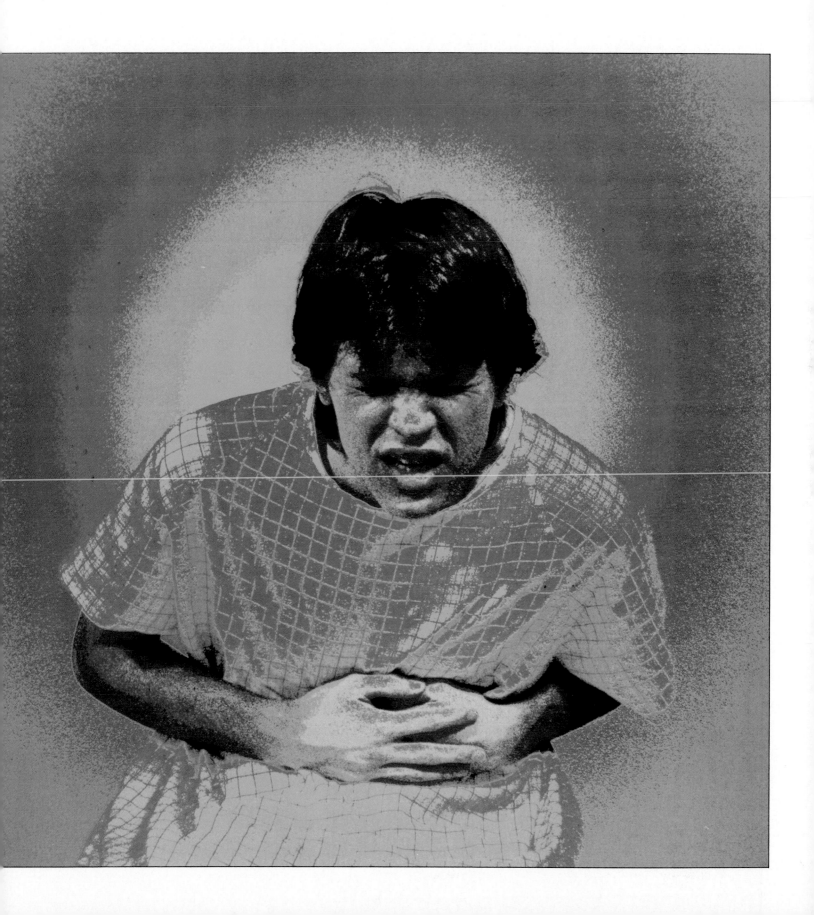

Pain management

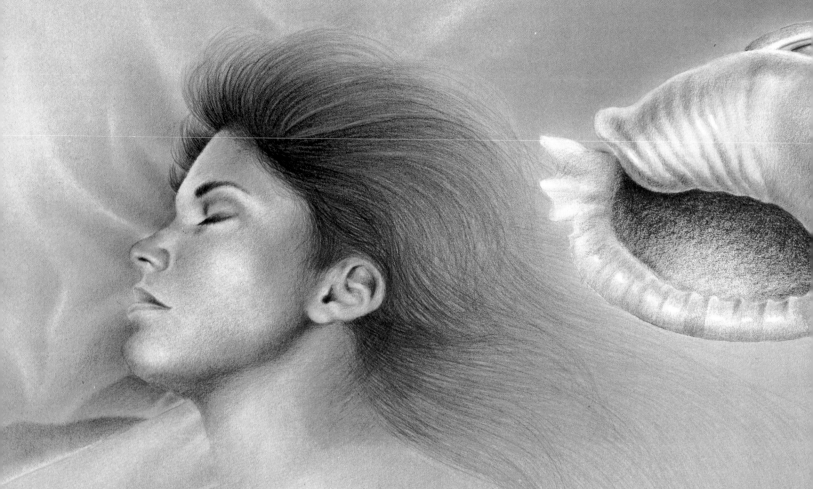

Using distraction to control pain

Distraction works well for brief episodes of pain caused, for example, by a dressing change, an injection, or turning in bed. Use any of the following distraction techniques, depending on which works best for your patient.

• Ask your patient to tell you about some interesting experience he's had.

• Have your patient's family obtain a tape recorder with headset and a cassette of the patient's favorite music. When he feels pain, have him turn on the music. He should close his eyes and concentrate only on the music, keeping time by tapping his foot or nodding his head. He may increase or decrease the music's volume as his pain increases or decreases.

What if your patient doesn't like music? He can listen instead to another type of recording; for example, of a sports event, or a comedy routine.

• If your patient likes to sing, ask him to do so, as he taps out the rhythm of a song. If he prefers, he can sing silently to himself, while mouthing the words and tapping out the rhythm.

• Try teaching your patient how to do rhythmic breathing. To do so, ask him to stare at an object as he first inhales and then exhales slowly. As he breathes, establish a rhythm for him by counting "in, 2, 3, 4; out, 2, 3, 4." Tell your patient to focus his attention on his breathing and accompany it with a mental image—either of air moving in and out of his lungs, or of any restful scene. Then, have him silently take over the count himself. But don't let him feel constrained by the rhythm you've set up. He should breathe at a comfortable rate.

You can vary the technique to provide for greater distraction by having the patient massage his arm or abdomen as he breathes. Or, have him inhale through his nose, and exhale through his mouth, or raise his head as he inhales and lower it as he exhales.

Using relaxation to control pain

Though distraction works well for acute, episodic pain, the patient can't keep it up indefinitely. So, for more enduring pain, try teaching your patient relaxation techniques. Deep relaxation, practiced for 20 to 40 minutes a day, will have a longer pain-relieving effect than distraction. Relaxation techniques tend to reduce anxiety, muscle tension pain, and fatigue. Their restorative qualities can enhance the effects of analgesics.

Given the increasing popularity of deep relaxation techniques for stress relief, your patient may already know one. If not, start him with some simple, natural relaxation practices, like sighing, yawning, or forming pleasant mental images.

More highly structured relaxation methods include meditation, yoga, self-hypnosis, breathing exercises, and biofeedback. Here, we'll explain how to teach your patient a breathing exercise. In performing this exercise, your patient may use the deep breathing method you taught him preoperatively.

• First, have him lie on his back in bed. Then, elevate his legs, with his knees bent. Place a pillow under his head. Tell him to breathe in and out slowly, as he did for the distraction exercise.

• Instruct him to listen closely to your voice. Then,

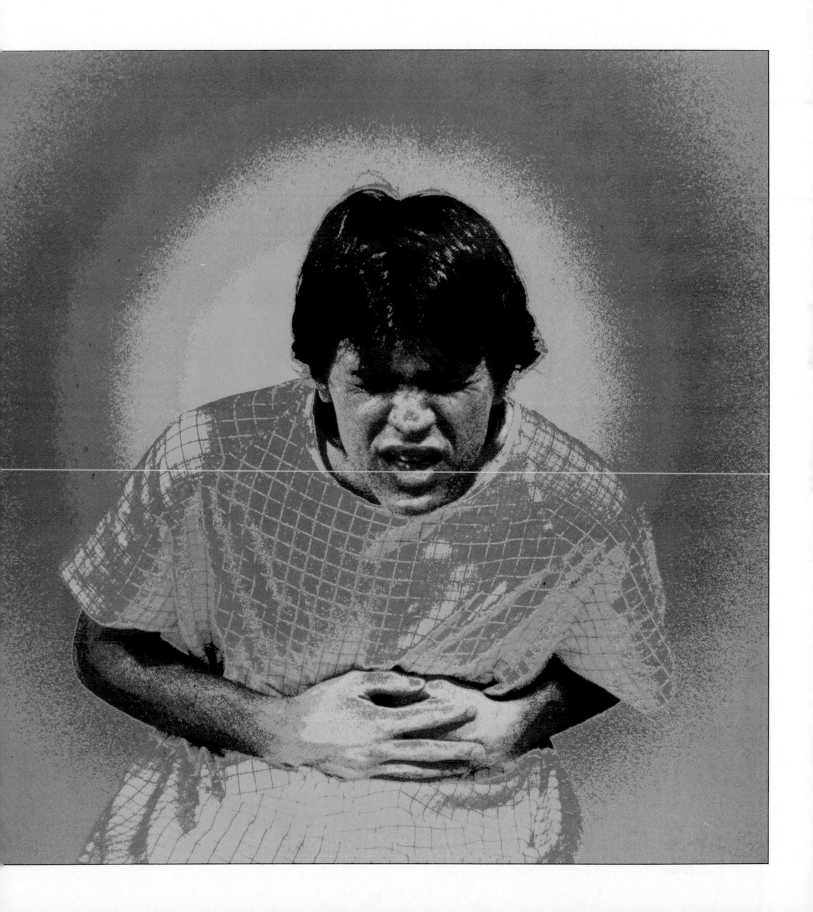

Pain management

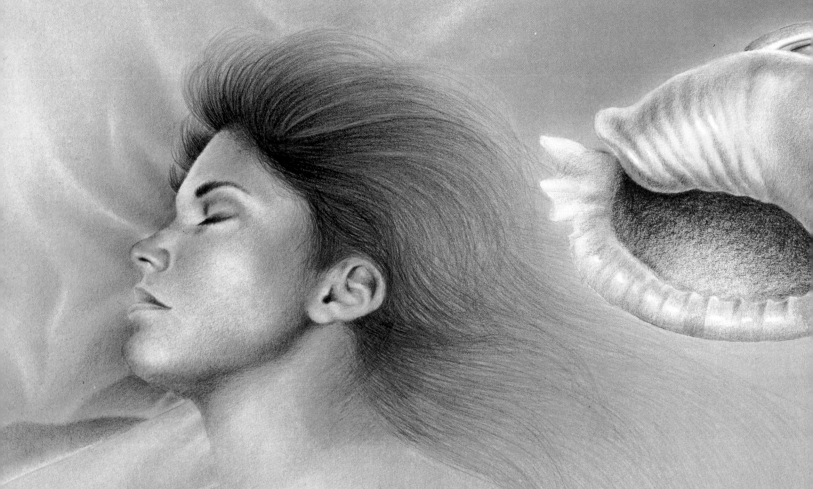

Using distraction to control pain

Distraction works well for brief episodes of pain caused, for example, by a dressing change, an injection, or turning in bed. Use any of the following distraction techniques, depending on which works best for your patient.

• Ask your patient to tell you about some interesting experience he's had.

• Have your patient's family obtain a tape recorder with headset and a cassette of the patient's favorite music. When he feels pain, have him turn on the music. He should close his eyes and concentrate only on the music, keeping time by tapping his foot or nodding his head. He may increase or decrease the music's volume as his pain increases or decreases.

What if your patient doesn't like music? He can listen instead to another type of recording; for example, of a sports event, or a comedy routine.

• If your patient likes to sing, ask him to do so, as he taps out the rhythm of a song. If he prefers, he can sing silently to himself, while mouthing the words and tapping out the rhythm.

• Try teaching your patient how to do rhythmic breathing. To do so, ask him to stare at an object as he first inhales and then exhales slowly. As he breathes, establish a rhythm for him by counting "in, 2, 3, 4; out, 2, 3, 4." Tell your patient to focus his attention on his breathing and accompany it with a mental image—either of air moving in and out of his lungs, or of any restful scene. Then, have him silently take over the count himself. But don't let him feel constrained by the rhythm you've set up. He should breathe at a comfortable rate.

You can vary the technique to provide for greater distraction by having the patient massage his arm or abdomen as he breathes. Or, have him inhale through his nose, and exhale through his mouth, or raise his head as he inhales and lower it as he exhales.

Using relaxation to control pain

Though distraction works well for acute, episodic pain, the patient can't keep it up indefinitely. So, for more enduring pain, try teaching your patient relaxation techniques. Deep relaxation, practiced for 20 to 40 minutes a day, will have a longer pain-relieving effect than distraction. Relaxation techniques tend to reduce anxiety, muscle tension pain, and fatigue. Their restorative qualities can enhance the effects of analgesics.

Given the increasing popularity of deep relaxation techniques for stress relief, your patient may already know one. If not, start him with some simple, natural relaxation practices, like sighing, yawning, or forming pleasant mental images.

More highly structured relaxation methods include meditation, yoga, self-hypnosis, breathing exercises, and biofeedback. Here, we'll explain how to teach your patient a breathing exercise. In performing this exercise, your patient may use the deep breathing method you taught him preoperatively.

• First, have him lie on his back in bed. Then, elevate his legs, with his knees bent. Place a pillow under his head. Tell him to breathe in and out slowly, as he did for the distraction exercise.

• Instruct him to listen closely to your voice. Then,

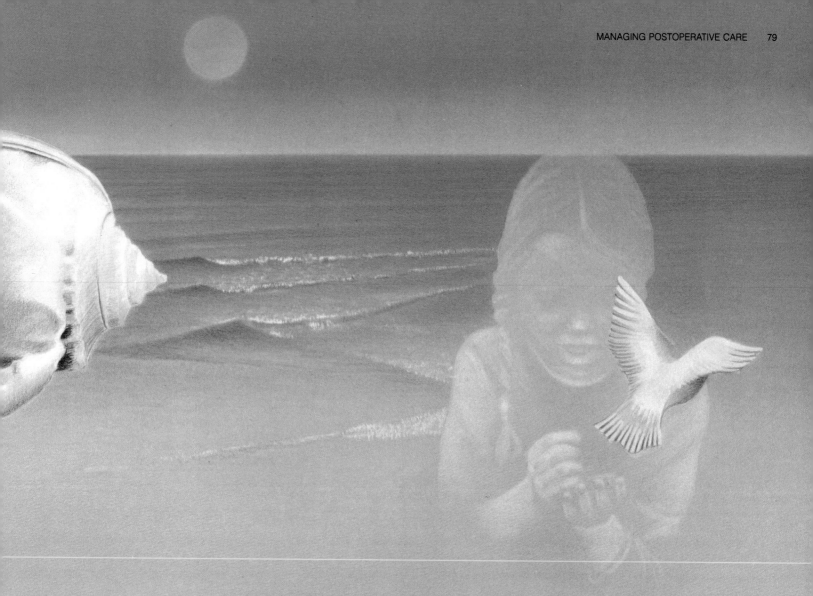

say: "Continue to breathe slowly and deeply, in a way that makes your abdomen expand and contract. Each time you exhale, feel yourself relaxing more. Notice how this makes you feel. You may feel weightless, pulsating, tingling, or heavy sensations.

"Mentally transport yourself to some pleasant location, such as the beach or park. Carefully note the details of sound, sight, smell, and touch associated with the place. When you're ready, end your relaxation exercise slowly, as you count to three. On the last count, remind yourself that you're awake, relaxed, and alert." *Note:* If your patient wants to sleep instead, have him end his relaxation exercise by telling himself that he's relaxed and ready to sleep.

Never limit yourself or your patient to one technique. A wide variety of activities will probably work, as long as each meets the following criteria:
• It uses the power of suggestion. (In other words, the patient believes the technique can work for him.)
• It distracts the patient's attention from his pain.
• It reduces the patient's anxiety level.
• It gives the patient a sense of control over pain.

Using cutaneous stimulation to control pain

For prevention or control of intense, lasting pain, try cutaneous stimulation: direct stimulation of the skin with cold or warm packs, menthol ointments, or contralateral stimulation. Consider the following suggestions. *Note:* Keep in mind that you may need a doctor's order to administer cutaneous stimulation. Check your hospital's policy.
• Cold packs may be ice bags, cold damp towels, or chilled reusable gel packs. Apply them directly to the painful area to slow the conduction of sensory impulses.
• Warm packs, water-filled heating pads or dry heating pads may provide temporary relief for some types of pain; for example, pain caused by vascular problems and joint disorders, such as bursitis.
• Menthol ointments induce sensations of warmth or coolness on the skin. They work well to relieve joint pain or pain associated with muscle tension. They may even help relieve visceral pain. Before using the ointment, rub a little on a small area of the patient's skin, to make sure it doesn't irritate the skin or cause an allergic reaction. Also, make sure the patient doesn't object to the menthol odor or sensation.

Important: Never apply a menthol ointment directly to patient's incision, or you could cause excoriation.
• Contralateral stimulation is cutaneous stimulation of the painful area's symmetrical counterpart. Use it when your patient has pain you can't reach or shouldn't touch. For example, if his *right* leg is in the cast, stimulate his left leg in precisely the same area of pain or irritation, with a cold pack or menthol ointment. Or, if his *right* foot throbs with incisional pain, stimulate his *left* foot. This technique also works for phantom pain.

Pain management

Learning about electronic pain control

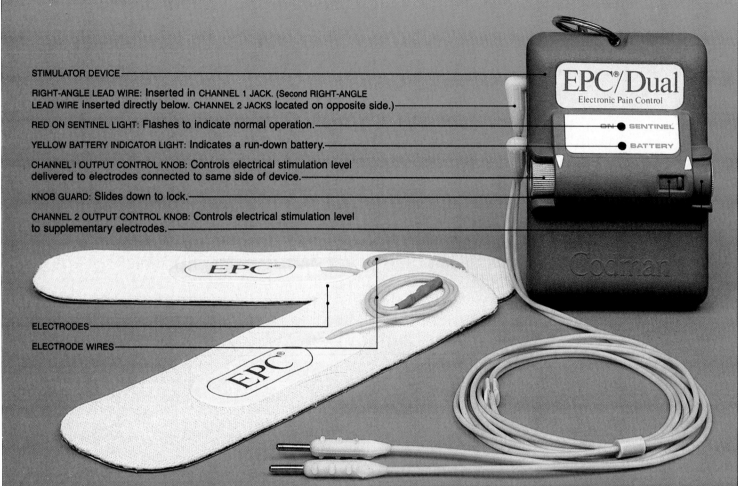

STIMULATOR DEVICE

RIGHT-ANGLE LEAD WIRE: Inserted in CHANNEL 1 JACK. (Second RIGHT-ANGLE LEAD WIRE inserted directly below. CHANNEL 2 JACKS located on opposite side.)

RED ON SENTINEL LIGHT: Flashes to indicate normal operation.

YELLOW BATTERY INDICATOR LIGHT: Indicates a run-down battery.

CHANNEL 1 OUTPUT CONTROL KNOB: Controls electrical stimulation level delivered to electrodes connected to same side of device.

KNOB GUARD: Slides down to lock.

CHANNEL 2 OUTPUT CONTROL KNOB: Controls electrical stimulation level to supplementary electrodes.

ELECTRODES

ELECTRODE WIRES

The side effects associated with narcotics and anesthetic drugs can trigger postop complications such as atelectasis, pneumonia, and paralytic ileus. So, any pain control method without serious side effects offers an advantage. For a patient with mild to moderate pain, the distraction or relaxation exercises we discussed on pages 78 and 79 may be adequate. But, a patient with moderate to severe pain might need a strong *external* stimulus to counteract the pain stimulus. In such a case, electronic pain control may help.

The EPC®/Dual Electronic Pain Control device (shown above) provides local transcutaneous electrical stimulation. It does so by transmitting a mild electrical current to nerves in the patient's skin, through electrodes applied externally near the surgical incision site. The mild electrical current probably relieves pain by overriding the transmission of pain impulses to the brain.

The only side effects the patient experiences are a mild tingling sensation and, possibly, local skin irritation under the electrodes. And the EPC/Dual system has another advantage: The patient actually can hold the device in his hand, so he can increase or decrease the amount of stimulation according to the degree of pain he feels. In itself, a sense of control over pain can be pain-relieving for a patient.

Electronic pain control seems to significantly reduce pain medication requirements in postoperative patients. In doing so, it reduces drug-associated side effects.

The EPC/Dual system isn't recommended for patients with myocardial disease or arrhythmias, or for patients with an indwelling line in the cardiac region (such as an internal or external pacemaker or any type of pulmonary artery line). In addition, its safe use for pregnant patients hasn't yet been proven, and it seems to work poorly for patients who have previously used narcotics.

When using this system, you must observe certain precautions. Keep in mind that this particular system's for external use only. In addition, never stimulate the eye area, the area over the carotid sinus nerves, or the area over the laryngeal or pharyngeal muscles. Doing so may interfere with critical nerve function.

If possible, teach your patient about electronic pain control preoperatively. This way, he'll accept and use the system more quickly after he's regained consciousness. If the system's effective for your patient, he may use the device throughout the period of postoperative pain.

Using the EPC®/Dual Electronic Pain Control system

1 *Here's how to use the EPC/Dual system:*
In the operating room, just before applying the dressing, the doctor places the system's two sterile electrodes on either side of the patient's suture line. Before doing so, he makes sure the application site is clean and dry. Then, he removes the paper backing from each electrode, and applies the electrode so that it's fully in contact with the skin.

The electrodes should be parallel to the patient's suture line, as shown below. For a long incision, or pain radiating over a large area, the doctor may apply a second pair of electrodes.

Next, the doctor covers the incision and electrodes with a dressing, making sure the electrodes' wires extend beyond the dressing.

Note: When the doctor applies the electrodes, he should transfer the sticker on the electrode package to the patient's chart. This way, all staff members will be aware that the patient is using the EPC/Dual system.

To attach the EPC/Dual stimulators in the recovery room, take the following steps.

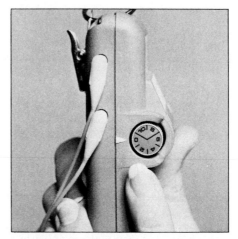

3 Now, turn on the OUTPUT CONTROL KNOB on the side you're using. Initially, set the control knob at a fairly low setting, such as level 2 or 3.

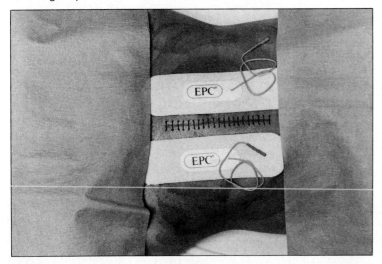

2 First, connect the pin (straight) end of a RIGHT-ANGLE LEAD WIRE to an ELECTRODE WIRE (see inset photo). Use a twisting motion to push the pin completely into the connector. Repeat this step for the second lead wire. Then, connect the lead wires' right-angled ends to the CHANNEL 1 JACKS, as shown in the larger photo. Insert the lead wires completely into the jacks.

Note: If the doctor's applied four electrodes, plug the second set of RIGHT-ANGLE LEAD WIRES into the CHANNEL 2 JACKS.

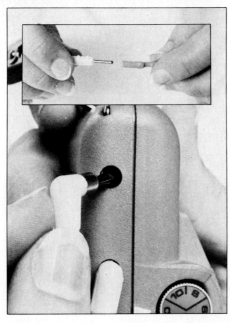

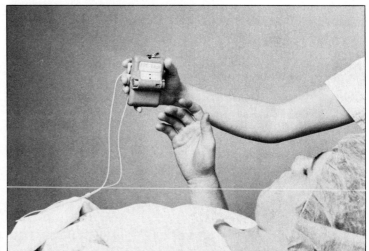

4 Then, give the patient the stimulator device, as the nurse is doing here, and allow him to find the level that provides pain relief. If your patient continually uses the higher levels (marked in red), remind him that a lower level may be sufficient. If he uses the higher levels because he's in severe pain, consider giving him analgesic medication.

Suppose your patient tells you the ON SENTINEL LIGHT has stopped flashing. First, turn the device off. Check to see if any wires are loose, disconnected, or damaged. Determine whether the wrong OUTPUT KNOB was turned on. Check the electrodes to see that they're undamaged and in good contact with the skin. If the electrodes become wet (as a result, for example, of excessive wound drainage), they may adhere poorly to the skin. (However, wet electrodes are not a safety hazard for the patient.) When you've identified the problem, correct it, if possible.

Note: The doctor may be responsible for replacing damaged or loosened electrodes. Check your hospital's policy.

The doctor may order that the stimulator be used continuously for 48 hours. Instruct your patient to notify you if he's not receiving adequate pain relief. If he does so, always check to make sure his device is operating properly before you administer any ordered medication.

Document in your nurses' notes the patient's use of the device and its effectiveness.

Ongoing care

Your patient's safely past the critical early postop period. Now, you'll gear your nursing care toward his early ambulation. The sooner he can ambulate, the less vulnerable he'll be to complications.

As you'll see, ongoing postop care includes a variety of procedures. Among the following photostories, charts, and illustrations, we'll detail how to logroll a patient who's undergone spinal surgery, make an occupied bed, apply restraints for patient safety, help your patient ambulate, and provide adequate nutrition.

Also, read these pages for tips on:
• using inflatable leggings to prevent thrombophlebitis.
• caring for a patient who needs restraints.
• teaching your patient postoperative range-of-motion exercises.

Turning in bed

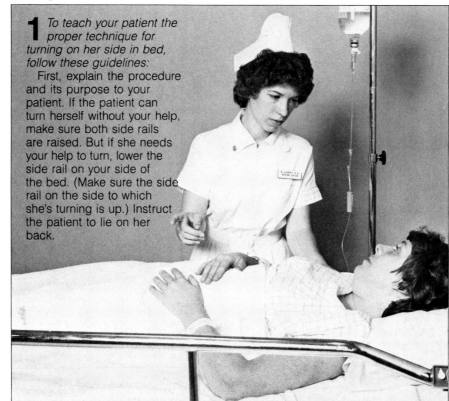

1 *To teach your patient the proper technique for turning on her side in bed, follow these guidelines:*
First, explain the procedure and its purpose to your patient. If the patient can turn herself without your help, make sure both side rails are raised. But if she needs your help to turn, lower the side rail on your side of the bed. (Make sure the side rail on the side to which she's turning is up.) Instruct the patient to lie on her back.

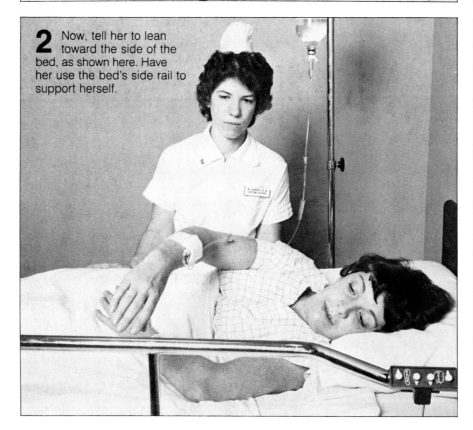

2 Now, tell her to lean toward the side of the bed, as shown here. Have her use the bed's side rail to support herself.

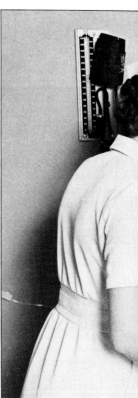

3 Next, have her shift her body weight to the side of her hip, rather than her buttock. Instruct her to dig her heels into the bed to lift her hips into position, and to use the side rail for support. *Note:* If your patient's body is at the edge of the bed, have her slide her shoulders and hips back to the bed's center.

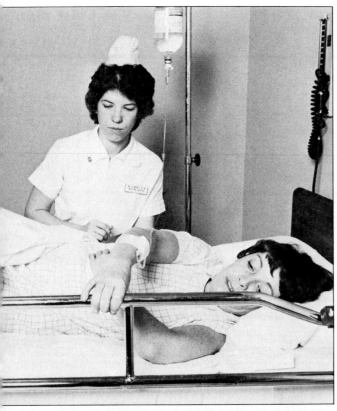

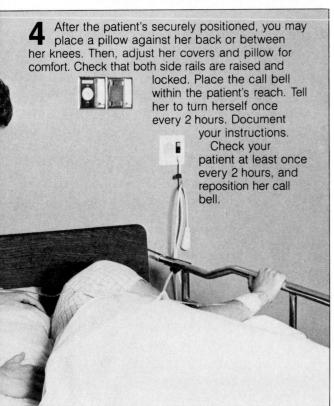

4 After the patient's securely positioned, you may place a pillow against her back or between her knees. Then, adjust her covers and pillow for comfort. Check that both side rails are raised and locked. Place the call bell within the patient's reach. Tell her to turn herself once every 2 hours. Document your instructions.

Check your patient at least once every 2 hours, and reposition her call bell.

Moving your patient safely

Whenever you reposition, turn, or transfer your patient, you risk straining your own musculoskeletal system. Apply good body-mechanics principles to help avoid injury. Keep these guidelines in mind:
• Before attempting to move your patient, assess his size and weight. Then, ask for help from your co-workers, if necessary.
• Carefully consider how you plan to move your patient. Discuss these plans with your co-workers.
• Clear obstacles from the area. Lock the bed's wheels and lower the side rail on your side.

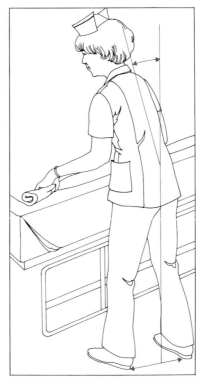

• Strengthen your support base by widening your stance, as shown in the above illustration. Keep one foot positioned slightly in front of the other.
• Before moving your patient, position his body as close to you as possible. Maneuver him into position by pushing rather than pulling, especially if he's heavy.
• To push your patient, stand close to his bed. Place one foot slightly in front of the other, front knee slightly bent. Keep most of your weight on your back foot. Place your palms on the patient's shoulder and hip closest to you.

Then, shifting your weight to your front foot, lean toward the patient and push gently, using your whole body.
• If you need to pull the patient toward you for any reason, assume the same position as for pushing. But this time, put most of your weight on your front foot. Slide your hands under the patient to the other side of his body. As you shift your weight to your rear foot, lean away from the patient, pulling with your body. Or, you may prefer this technique: Roll the drawsheet close to the patient's body and pull with it.

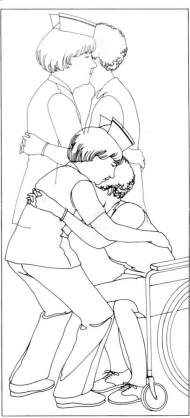

• When moving a patient, keep your back and upper body straight. Always use your major leg muscles rather than your back muscles for repositioning, as the nurse is doing in the illustration above.

Lower your body to the patient's level by bending your knees, not by leaning over from the waist. Shift your weight to your front foot. Lift by straightening your knees and hips, keeping your upper body straight.

Ongoing care

How to logroll a patient after spinal surgery

1 *Caring for a patient who's had a laminectomy? If you are, you'll have to move him from a supine to a side-lying position every 2 hours, keeping his spine immobilized throughout the procedure. If he has a folded drawsheet (turning sheet) under him, ask a coworker to help you perform the logrolling technique shown here.*

First, obtain three pillows. Then, making sure the bed is flat, raise it to a comfortable working height. Stand at the side of the bed that you want to turn your patient away from. Then, lower the side rail on that side of the bed.

Explain the procedure to your patient and remove his top covers, as the nurse is doing here.

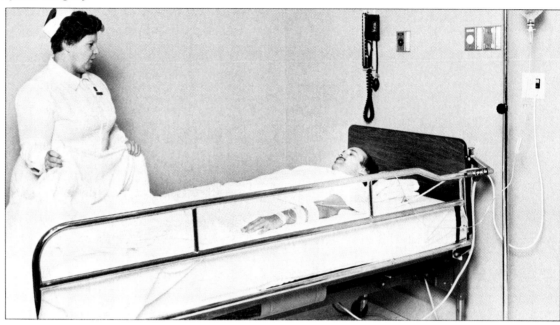

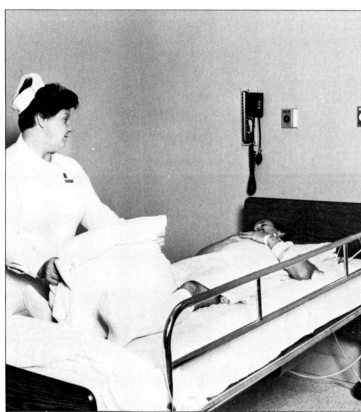

2 Now, position your patient properly. To do so, have him bend his elbows and place his hands on his chest. Also, ask him to straighten his legs, keeping his feet together. If he's not strong enough to do this, place a pillow between his legs. Instruct him to maintain this position throughout the procedure. (You don't want him to bend his body at his waist or hips while you're turning him.)

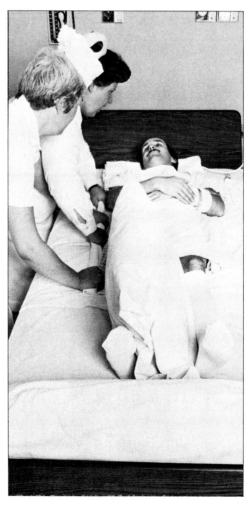

3 Now, ask a coworker to help you roll up the turning sheet. Roll it tightly against the patient, as the nurses are doing here. (Notice the crossed-arm technique they're using.) Steadily pull the patient toward you, if necessary, to allow enough room for you to turn him.

4 Place two pillows against the side rail, to cushion the patient when he turns. Then, instruct him to reach for the side rail as you and your co-worker turn him. To promote muscle relaxation during the procedure, also instruct him to deep breathe.

On a predetermined signal, use the turning sheet to roll the patient on his side. Take care to keep his body properly aligned.

While your co-worker places the patient's legs in a comfortable position, support the patient with your hands, as shown here.

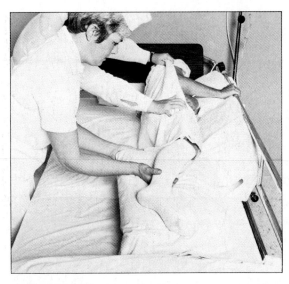

5 Then, remove the pillows against the side rail, and place them against the patient's back for support, as the nurses are doing here.

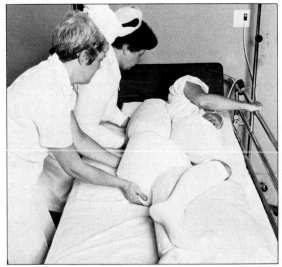

6 Reposition the pillow under the patient's head, so he's comfortable. If you haven't done so already, place a pillow between his legs, to prevent pressure sores. Then, replace his top covers, and raise the side rail. After making sure both side rails are locked, place the call bell within the patient's reach. Finally, document the position change in your nurses' notes.

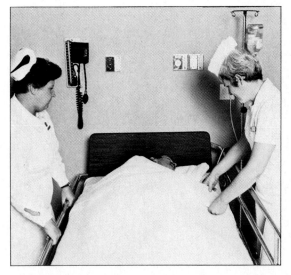

Learning about the Athrombic™ pump

Is your patient restricted to long-term bed rest? If so, the doctor may order the Jobst® Athrombic™ pump and inflatable leggings to help prevent deep-vein thrombosis in your patient.

This electrically-powered pump automatically inflates leggings that are applied to your patient's calves. The leggings provide external pneumatic compression of the capillaries and small veins in the calves. This forces blood into the larger leg veins, accelerating blood flow so the blood doesn't pool and clot.

Patients who are at high risk of developing deep-vein thrombosis, and who would benefit from the leggings, include:
• patients who've had neurosurgery
• patients who've had open urologic surgery
• patients with spinal cord injuries
• patients who've had a myocardial infarction
• surgical patients over age 40.

Doctors may prefer inflatable leggings to antiembolism stockings for patients who'll have restricted mobility over a long time period. But, leggings may not be practical for patients who can walk, because electricity is needed to power the equipment.

If the doctor orders inflatable leggings for your patient, try to apply them before surgery. If you can't, apply the leggings as soon as possible after surgery.

Important: Don't apply the leggings if your patient has been immobilized for more than 24 hours; the external pneumatic compression may move an already-formed clot.

Also, don't apply leggings if your patient has had leg surgery, has a leg infection, a pulmonary embolism, or is in the acute stages of inflammatory phlebitis.

If the doctor orders inflatable leggings for your patient, be sure to take these special precautions:
• Remove them once every 8 hours for at least an hour to assess your patient's skin. Cleanse the patient's legs as well.
• Check the leggings periodically to make sure they fit properly. They should fit snugly, but shouldn't restrict blood flow to the patient's feet and toes when inflated or deflated. If the leggings are applied properly and fit snugly, they will quickly begin supplying the necessary external pneumatic compression.

Ongoing care

Using the Athrombic™ pump

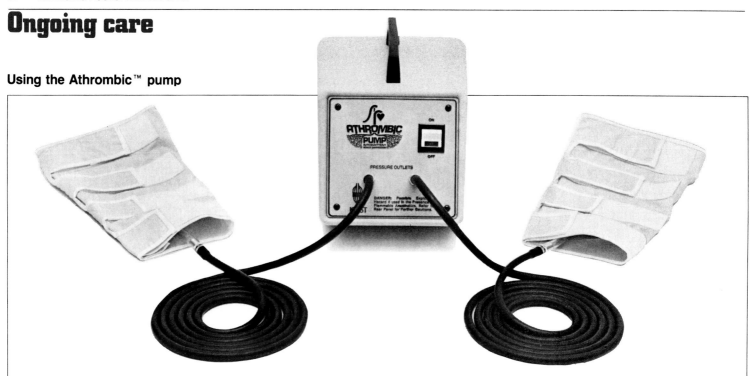

1 *Ruth Merriwether, a 42-year-old legal secretary, is recovering from a craniotomy, and will temporarily be on bed rest. During that time, her doctor wants her to wear inflatable leggings. Since she's your patient, you'll have to apply them. Do you know how?*

If you're using the Athrombic pump and inflatable leggings, follow the steps in this photostory:
Gather the equipment pictured here: two wrap-around inflatable leggings, two rubber air-delivery tubes, and the Athrombic compression pump.

2 Tell your patient how the leggings work and why they're needed. Explain that she'll probably have to wear them until she's no longer on bed rest.

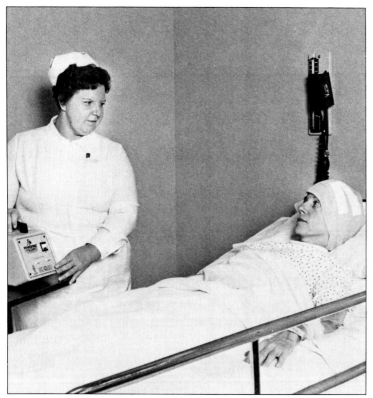

3 Place the inflatable bladder of one legging beneath the patient's calf, with the legging's narrow end near her ankle. Then, wrap the legging around her calf and use the Velcro® straps to secure it, as shown. Make sure the straps fasten on top of the patient's calf. Follow the same procedure with the other legging.

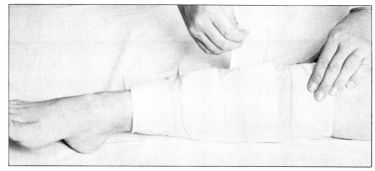

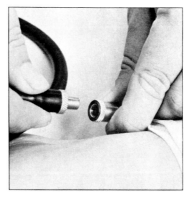

4 Insert the metal fitting at the end of each rubber air delivery tube into the metal fitting on each legging, as shown.

5 Place the unattached ends of the rubber tubes over the pressure outlets on the pump, as shown here. Next, plug the machine into a properly-grounded electrical outlet. Place the machine on the floor at the foot of the patient's bed, taking care to position the cord where no one can trip over it. *Note:* Never leave the pump under the patient's bed, where it may become damaged as the bed is raised or lowered.

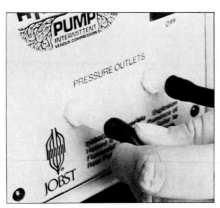

6 Set the power button to the ON position. The Athrombic pump will automatically supply 45 mm Hg for 15 seconds out of every minute to inflate the leggings. *Note:* Several inflation cycles may occur before the leggings are fully inflated.

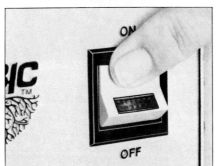

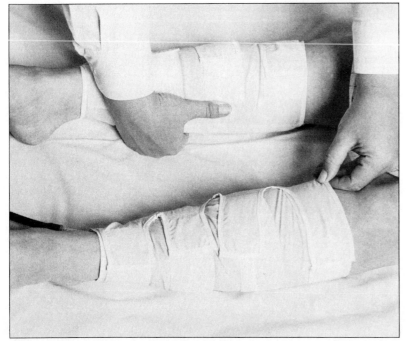

7 Check the leggings periodically to make sure they fit properly. Remove and reapply them, if necessary.
To discontinue treatment, set the power button to the OFF position. Unplug the machine. Disconnect the air delivery tubes from the leggings. Allow the leggings to deflate. Then, remove them. Assure your patient that any marks left on her skin from the leggings will disappear in about 30 minutes. Document what you've done in your nurses' notes.

Helping your patient with personal care

Marybeth Warner, a 40-year-old accountant, is recovering satisfactorily from a partial colectomy. Her condition is such that she can now provide her own mouth care and bathe herself. You'll want to help her.

To do this, first explain exactly how much you want her to do. Then, assist her, as follows:
• Provide your patient with the mouth-care equipment she'll need: an emesis basin, towel, toothbrush and toothpaste, mouthwash, denture cup (if needed), dental floss, and a cup of water. When she's finished using them, remove the equipment.
• Next, obtain bath equipment, including a wash basin, soap, washcloth, towel, bath blanket, and personal toilet articles such as deodorant, comb and hairbrush, slippers, and clean gown. Place the equipment on an overbed table.
• Provide privacy for the patient by screening her bed or closing the door to her room.
• Help her sit upright on the side of the bed. Remove her antiembolism stockings, if she's wearing any, and put on her slippers.

For stability, her feet should touch the floor. If they don't, give her a padded footstool to rest them on. *Note:* If your patient can't sit on the side of the bed for any reason, place her in a semi-Fowler's position.
• Now, fold back the sheets so they're out of her way. Spread a bath blanket over her lap. Then, place the overbed table with the equipment on it within her reach.
• Fill the basin with *warm* water, and place it on the overbed table.
• Help the patient out of her gown. Adjust any drainage tubes or other equipment as necessary. Take advantage of this opportunity to observe her for any fatigue, pain, bleeding, or other signs of discomfort.
• Caution her to wash carefully around drainage tubes and dressings, to avoid wetting them.
• Instruct her to wash her perineal area last. Ask her not to use this washcloth again after she's washed her perineal area.
• If all's well, leave her alone to bathe in privacy. But, be sure that you make arrangements to return at a set time. The patient will feel reassured if she knows exactly when you'll be back to help her.
• When you return to your patient, ask how much of her bath she was able to complete. Then, obtain fresh warm water and a clean washcloth. Finish washing and drying those areas she couldn't reach, such as her feet and back.
• Complete the patient's bath by giving her a backrub and applying lotion, if the patient wishes. If your patient uses deodorant, help her apply it, if necessary. Then, help her into a clean gown or pajamas. Apply clean antiembolism stockings, if appropriate.
• Remove the bath equipment from the overbed table. Discard soiled linen in a laundry hamper. Clean any reusable bath equipment and store it.
• Then, hand her a comb and brush, so she can care for her hair. Make sure the mirror on her overbed table is positioned so she can use it.
• When she's finished, help her get comfortable once again. Urge her to rest if she's tired.
• Document your observations in your nurses' notes.

Ongoing care

Giving your patient a bed bath

1 *Following your patient's surgery, encourage him to resume normal activity, including bathing, as soon as possible. Until then, you'll bathe him yourself. Here's how:*
Obtain the equipment shown here: a wash basin, soap, washcloths and towels, bath blanket, cotton-tipped applicators, lotion, clean gown, and mouth care articles. Also obtain a comb or brush, and any other toilet articles your patient uses (such as deodorant). Since bathing the patient provides a good opportunity to change the bed, obtain a clean set of bed linens, too.

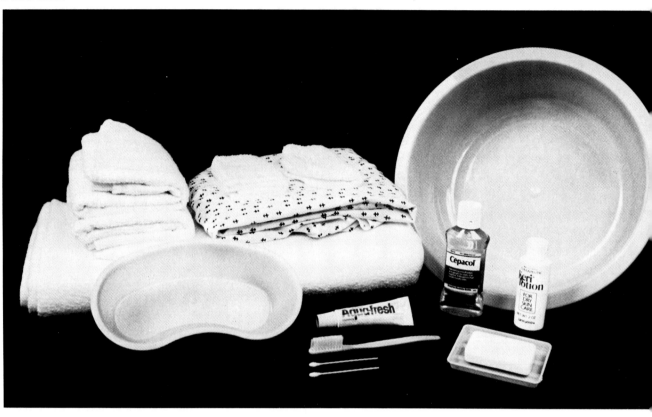

2 Help your patient perform mouth care just before you give him his bath. Then, if possible, position your patient on his back. Elevate the bed to a comfortable working height. Explain the procedure to him.

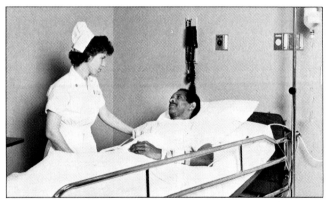

3 Place the bath blanket over the patient, on top of the covers. Ask him to hold the top edge of the bath blanket, as he's doing here. Then, pulling from the foot of the bed, remove the covers. Discard them in a linen hamper, or according to hospital policy.

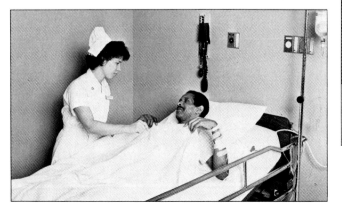

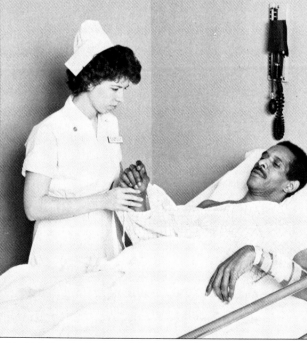

4 Fold back the bath blanket, and remove the patient's gown. Cover him again with the blanket. Don't forget to remove his antiembolism stockings, if he's wearing any.

5 Now, fill the wash basin with very warm water. (Remember, your patient will probably find lukewarm bath water unpleasant.) Place the filled basin on an easy-to-reach surface; for example, on the overbed table.

[Inset] Next, wrap the washcloth around your hand, as shown, tucking in all loose ends. Moisten the washcloth with warm water. Squeeze out excess water. (If your patient usually washes his face with soap, apply soap to the washcloth, too.)

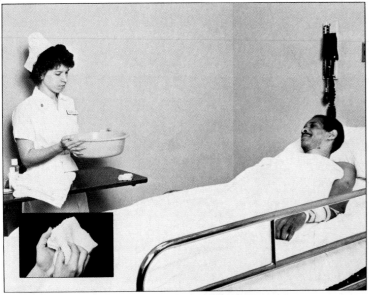

6 Gently wash the patient's face. Then, ask the patient to close his eyes. Wash each eyelid, beginning at the inside corner. Immediately rinse and dry his eyelids; then do the same to the rest of his face.

Gently wash, rinse, and dry the patient's ears and neck. Then, use cotton-tipped applicators to clean his auricles.

Important: Never clean inside the ear canals.

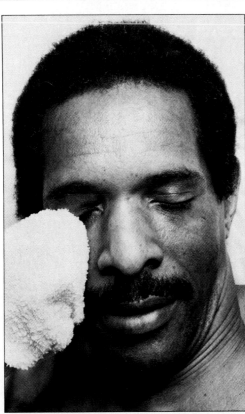

7 Place a towel on top of the bath blanket and place the patient's arm on top of the towel. Beginning with his hand, wash his hand and arm (including his underarm). As you work, take this opportunity to help your patient perform range-of-motion exercises. Rinse and dry his hand and arm with a clean towel. Apply deodorant, if your patient wishes. Repeat the procedure for the other hand, arm, and underarm. Remove the towel you placed on top of the bath blanket.

During this portion of the bath, consider immersing the patient's hands in water. He'll find this soothing. Dry his hands afterward.

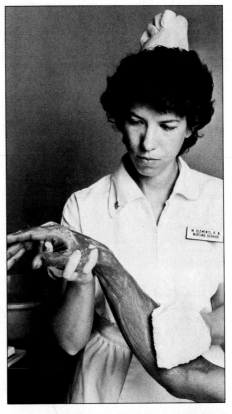

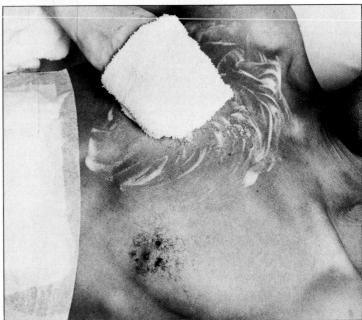

8 Then, fold back the bath blanket, and wash your patient's chest and abdomen. If your patient has an abdominal incision, take special care to wash around the dressing without wetting it. Rinse and dry his skin; then, cover him again with the bath blanket.

Important: If your patient's a woman, take special care to wash under her breasts. Then, thoroughly dry her skin.

Ongoing care

Giving your patient a bed bath continued

9 Obtain fresh, warm water. Fold back the bath blanket to expose the patient's legs, and lay a towel under his legs to protect the bed linen. Bathe each of his legs in the same way you bathed his arms. Support his legs, when necessary.

[Inset] If possible, soak his feet (one at a time, or together) in the warm water. Remember to dry them afterward.

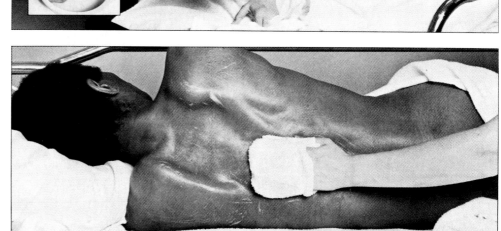

10 Now, prepare to wash the patient's back. Again, obtain fresh, warm water. Lower the head of the bed so the patient's flat (unless the patient's uncomfortable in this position). Ask the patient to roll away from you, so he's lying on his side, as shown here. (Remember, by encouraging him to roll himself, you increase his mobility. However, help him roll, if necessary.) To protect the bed, lay a towel behind his back. Wash, rinse, and dry his back, including his buttocks, and remove the towel.

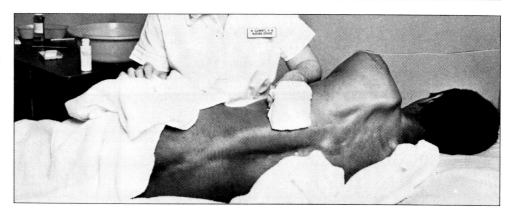

11 Now, ask the patient to roll slightly toward you, so you can wash the rest of his back (including the portion of his buttocks that was inaccessible before.) Rinse and dry his skin. Remove the towel.

12 Again, ask the patient to roll to his left side, so you can easily reach his rectal area. Replace the towel behind his buttocks, and wash his rectal area. Dry his skin, remove the towel, and discard the washcloth in a linen hamper, or according to hospital policy.

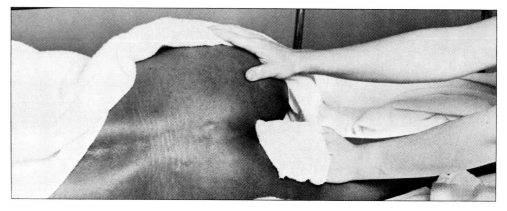

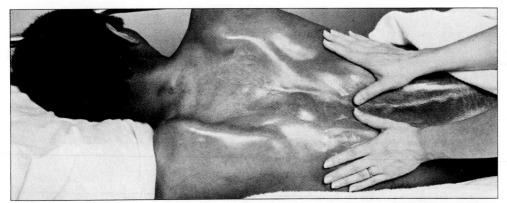

13 Now, while the patient remains on his left side, massage his back and buttocks. For your patient's comfort, warm the lotion bottle with your hands. Then, apply lotion and pat it dry with a towel, if necessary.

Change the bottom linens on the bed, following the procedure detailed in the next photostory. During the procedure (while the patient's repositioned on his right side), remember to massage the other side of his back and buttocks, and to apply lotion.

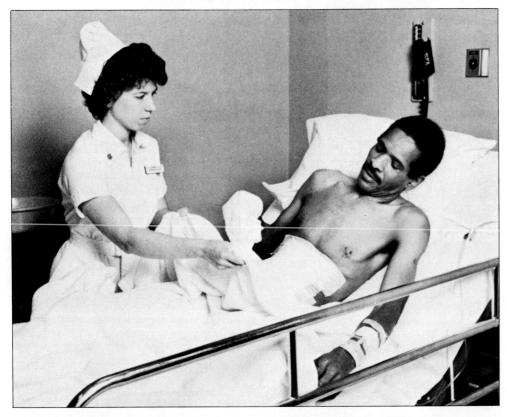

14 Position the patient on his back, and raise the head of the bed to a position that's comfortable for him. Again, obtain fresh, warm water and give the patient a clean washcloth and the soap. If he's able, ask him to perform his own perineal care. Because this care is so personal, most patients prefer to perform it themselves. But if your patient isn't able to do so, wash the area for him. *Note:* Instruct your patient to cleanse the perineal area from the front to the back, to avoid spreading rectal bacteria. If your patient is uncircumcised, tell him to retract his foreskin and gently cleanse the head of his penis. (If your patient's a female, instruct her to pay special attention to cleansing the folds of skin.) Then, make sure the perineal area is rinsed and dried thoroughly.

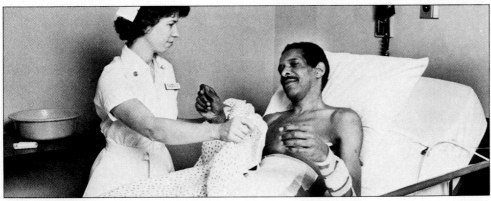

15 Help the patient into a clean gown or pajamas, and apply a clean pair of antiembolism stockings, if appropriate.

Place clean bed linens over the bath blanket. Then, as the patient holds the top of the bed linens, remove the bath blanket by pulling it out from the foot of the bed. Tuck in the top linens at the foot of the bed.

Dispose of all equipment and provide for any other personal hygiene care. For example, you may shave a male patient, if he's unable to shave himself. Also, give him the comb, so he can care for his hair.

Document any problems you noticed; for example, developing pressure sores.

Ongoing care

Making an occupied bed

1 *Today, good nursing care emphasizes early ambulation rather than prolonged bed rest. But, depending on your patient's condition and the type of surgery she's had, she may require several days of bed rest. So, you may have to make her bed while she's in it. Here's what to do:*
First, obtain clean linen, including two sheets, two drawsheets, pillow cases, blanket, and bed-saver pads.

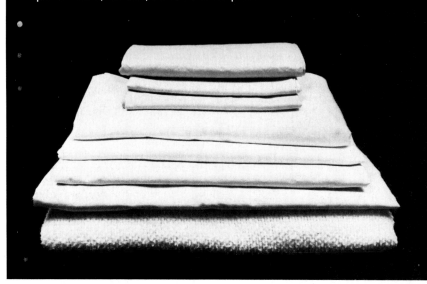

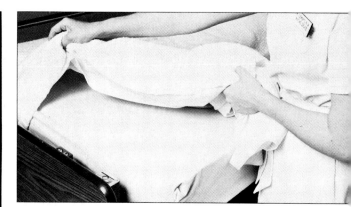

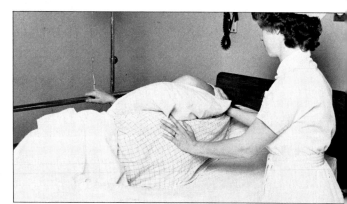

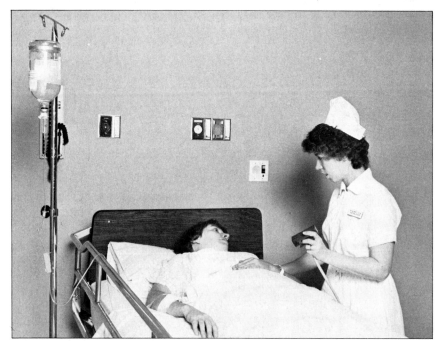

2 Explain the procedure to the patient and suggest ways she can help. Make sure the side rail on the opposite side of the bed is raised. Then, lower the bed's head, if necessary, and raise the bed to your waist level. *Note:* When repositioning your patient, consider the location of her wound. Your main concern is to make her as comfortable as possible.

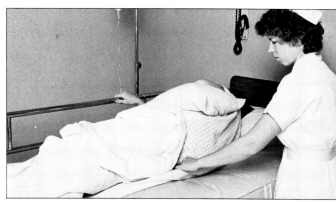

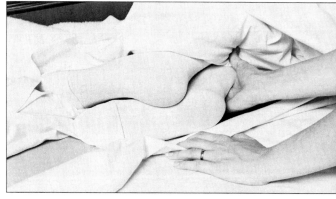

3 Remove any extra pillows. Then, loosen the top sheet. To provide privacy for your patient, use the top sheet as a drape.

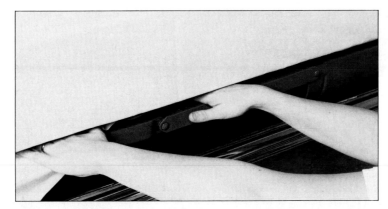

4 Give your patient a pillow for splinting her wound. Then, consider the side you want your patient to lie on after the procedure, according to her turning schedule. For example, if you want her on her left side, begin by positioning her on her right side. This way, when you finish the procedure, she'll be lying on her left side.

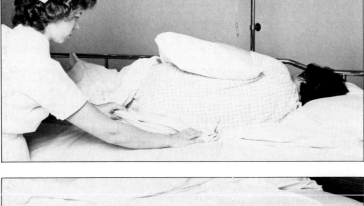

5 Loosen the bottom sheets on the side you're working on. Roll them up very tightly with the folded drawsheet (turning sheet), rolling toward the bed's center. Make the roll as small as possible. Tuck the roll under the patient's back.

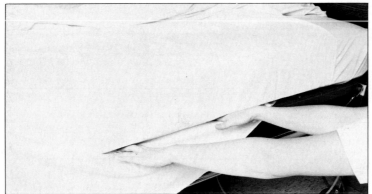

6 Now, place the clean bottom sheet lengthwise on the near half of the bed. Center it so that both sides unfold on that side of the bed. Roll half of the bottom sheet to the bed's center. Tuck it under the patient.

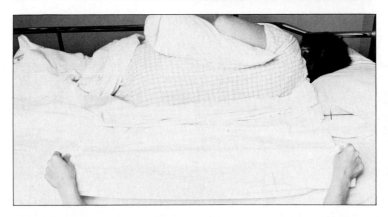

7 Tuck in the remaining half of the bottom sheet at the head and sides of the bed, smoothing out any wrinkles.

8 Place a bed-saver pad on the bed, centering it midway between the head and foot of the bed. Tuck the bed-saver pad under the patient, as shown here.
Note: If necessary (for example, if the patient's surgical wound is on an extremity), place a second bed-saver pad under the area of expected drainage.

9 Cover the bed-saver pad with a drawsheet. Roll up the other half of the drawsheet and tuck it under the patient. Tuck in the near side of the drawsheet, as shown here.

10 Next, fold a drawsheet in half to make a turning sheet. Place the turning sheet over the drawsheet. Roll up the turning sheet's opposite half and place it under the patient. Fanfold the edge of the sheet that hangs over the bed. Let it rest on the bed's edge.
Nursing tip: If you place a bath blanket under the patient and over the rolled-up sheets, you'll protect them from drainage or moisture when she rolls over.

Ongoing care

Making an occupied bed continued

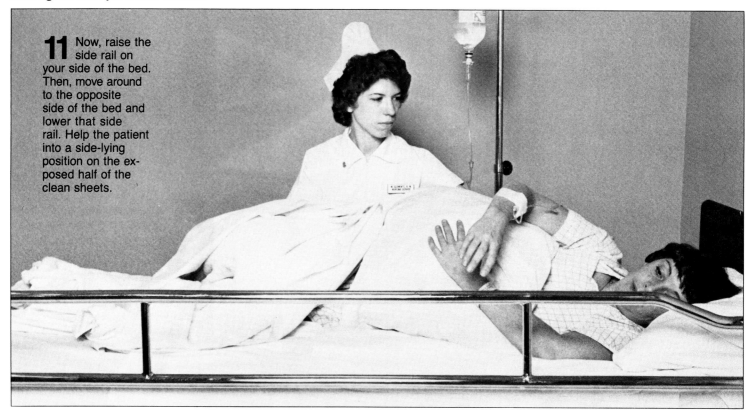

11 Now, raise the side rail on your side of the bed. Then, move around to the opposite side of the bed and lower that side rail. Help the patient into a side-lying position on the exposed half of the clean sheets.

12 Then, remove the soiled bottom sheets from the bed. Place them in the linen hamper immediately. Never put them on the floor or furniture. Also, avoid touching your uniform with the soiled sheets.

Next, unroll the near half of the bottom sheet and drawsheets. Pull the sheets tightly to eliminate wrinkles, and tuck them in under the mattress.

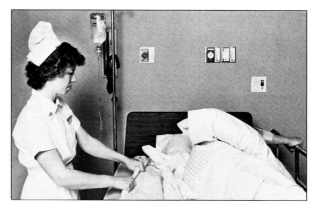

13 Help the patient into a comfortable position, according to her turning schedule. Then, center a clean top sheet on top of the soiled top linens. Unfold it to each side. Working from the foot of the bed, have the patient hold the top edge of the clean sheet while you pull off the soiled linens. Immediately place the soiled linens in the linen hamper.

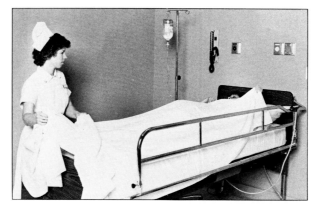

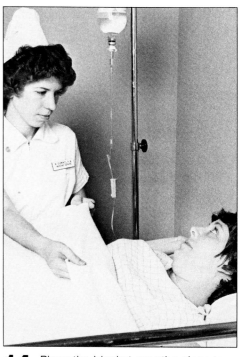

14 Place the blanket over the clean top sheet. Fold the sheet back over the blanket and form a cuff, as the nurse has done here.

15 Allowing about 4" to 6" (10.2 to 15.2 cm) of slack in the top covers, tuck them in at the foot of the bed. Miter the corners at the foot of the bed, on both sides. But don't tuck in the sides of the top covers.

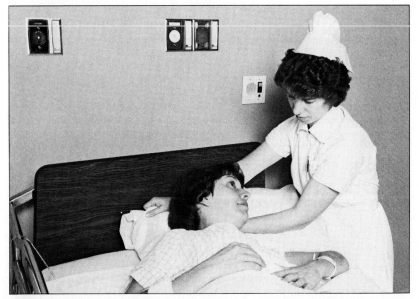

16 Gently remove the pillow from under the patient's head. Remove the pillowcase, and place it in the linen hamper. Replace the pillowcase with a new one, and place the pillow under the patient's head. Replace pillowcases on any other pillows used for positioning. Before leaving the patient, check that all tubes and drains are patent. Ask the patient if she's comfortable. Lower the bed and check that both side rails are securely locked in the raised position. Place the call bell within the patient's reach.

Document any observations in your nurses' notes.

Does your patient need restraints?

Suppose your patient's extremely agitated or disoriented. Consider the possibility that, for his safety, you may need to apply restraints.

The following guidelines will help you decide whether your patient needs restraints. But remember, as a rule, you aren't permitted to apply (or remove) restraints without a doctor's order. In addition, many hospitals have specific procedures for checking and removing restraints. Learn your hospital's policy, and follow it.

To determine whether your patient needs restraints, assess the extent of his confusion. A mildly confused elderly patient may benefit more from your attentive, systematic efforts to reorient him than from restraints. In fact, restraining him may only *increase* his agitation. But, in some instances, a patient may need to be restrained for his own protection, until he achieves self-control.

To evaluate your patient's confusion, check his orientation to time and place. Ask him simple questions about where he is, why he's in the hospital, and what day it is. Phrase the questions clearly and try to slant them to your patient's cultural background. Take into account any special handicaps the patient has communicating; for example, lack of fluency in English, a hearing or sight impediment, or preexisting memory problems. (Also, keep in mind that your patient's speech may sound garbled if his dentures have been removed.)

If, in addition to being confused, your patient's agitated and combative, he'll probably need restraints. The same holds true if he seems to be hallucinating or if he attempts to leave the bed without your assistance.

Let's say you've assessed your patient carefully, and you're certain that he *does* need restraints. As a rule, obtain a doctor's order for the restraints *before* you apply them. However, if you're facing a full-fledged emergency, you may have to apply the restraints first and *then* get the doctor's order (as soon as possible).

Next, try to overcome your patient's resistance. Even though he's disoriented, you owe him an explanation of why you're imposing the restraints. State gently, but firmly, that he's upset, confused, and out of control. Explain that you must apply the restraints for *his* protection, so that he won't hurt himself. Reassure him that you'll remove the restraints as soon as possible. If his family is present, reassure them too, and explain the purpose of the restraints.

Before applying the restraints, think through how you'll do it and if you'll need help from co-workers. Agree upon each staff member's role beforehand; for example, who will hold which part of the patient's body. Plan what you'll do if he offers resistance. You may need a doctor's order to sedate him. *Important:* If your patient's on bed rest, tie the restraint to the bed frame—*never* the side rail.

To find out more about restraints, study the chart on the following page.

Ongoing care

Nurses' guide to restraints

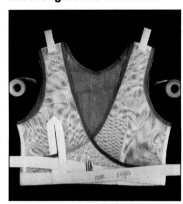

Type and description	Indications	Nursing considerations
Jacket restraint A vest with shoulder loops and straps. May be fastened at waist only, or at waist and shoulders for greater security.	For a confused, but not seriously agitated patient, to keep her from leaving her bed or chair	• Use extra straps through the shoulder loops for greater security and to keep the patient from sitting up or sliding down in bed. Tie them to the bed frame at the top of the bed and place a pillow over them. • When using the jacket restraint in a chair, bring the straps up over the back of the chair. Then, tie them to the chair's frame. • Tie the straps securely, but not too tightly. Doing otherwise could alter the patient's spinal cord alignment, or inhibit her chest and lung expansion.

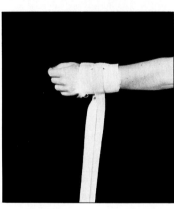

Limb restraint A padded holder with Velcro closures. Designed with extra loop to ensure a comfortable fit without the need for constant adjustments.	For a patient who's disoriented or confused because of anesthetic (or other medication) effects	• To tie restraint properly, first put each strap through the loop from the opposite direction. Tie the straps in a knot around the loop. Then, wrap the straps around each other in a crisscross pattern until they form one strap. Tie the end to the bed frame. • Tie the restraint toward the foot of the bed rather than the head. Doing otherwise would allow the patient to increase his range of motion by bending his elbow. • Check the restrained limb's range of motion. Make sure the patient can't reach any equipment, such as an I.V. pole. (If necessary, consider restraining the opposite limb, too.)

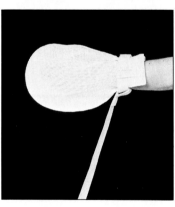

Mitten restraint A translucent mitt with extra strap for attaching to bed frame. Also available with rigid palm. The translucent mitt allows you to observe the patient's hand for alterations in skin color.	For a mildly agitated patient who may yank I.V. tubes or tamper with drainage equipment	• Don't allow the restraint to bind or bend the patient's fingers. Obtain the natural position of partial hand flexion by placing a large roll of dressings or a rolled washcloth in the patient's palm. • Consider using the extra strap to further restrain his hand. With the mitt alone, the patient may still be able to damage any equipment he has.

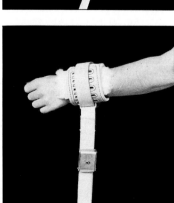

Leather restraint A fur-lined leather limb holder with key lock. May be applied to patient's arms or legs.	For a strong, violent patient who is disoriented or agitated	• When necessary, don't hesitate to use this restraint instead of a cloth restraint. A strong patient may easily tear loose from cloth restraints.

Caring for a restrained patient

You might think that a restrained patient requires little care. But he needs your close attention. By restraining your patient, you've made him more dependent on you. Instead of feeding himself, for example, he'll rely on you to do it. If he's struggling against his restraints, closely monitor him to keep him from untying them or entangling himself. Also, watch for any developing abrasions or bruises.

Consider the following as necessary steps in performing care for a restrained patient:
• Check pulses distal to the restraint frequently. Every hour, check the area under the restraint for abrasions or bruising. In addition, check the entire limb for position, alignment, and circulation.
• Every 2 hours, loosen the restraint and help the patient perform range-of-motion exercises for the affected limb or limbs. Massage his buttocks, heels, elbows, and any other pressure points.
• Reposition him every 2 hours. Never assume he must lie only on his back.
• Give him a bedpan or escort him to the bathroom at least once every 2 hours.
• Periodically assess your patient's confusion to determine whether he still needs the restraint.

When should you ask the doctor for an order to remove the restraint? As early as possible; for example, when your patient demonstrates orientation, self-control, and cooperation. Then, remove each restraint cautiously—one extremity at a time—assessing your patient's behavior as you proceed. Provide your patient with emotional support. He'll need reassurance that his behavior is now acceptable.

Document what you've done in your nurses' notes.

Ambulating your patient

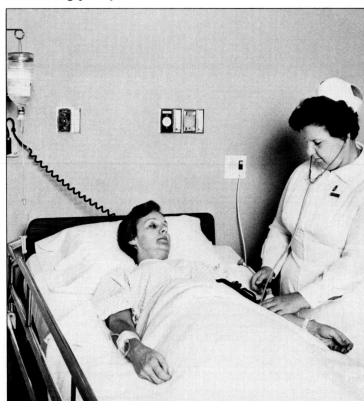

1 *Your patient returned from the recovery room at 4 p.m. The doctor's ordered you to ambulate her at 9 p.m. What steps should you take? Read the following photostory to find out.*

At 8:45 p.m. (or shortly before you plan to ambulate the patient), document her vital signs. If her vital signs are unstable, or if you see any signs or symptoms of complications, don't proceed without notifying the doctor.

Note: For your patient's comfort, plan to help her ambulate 15 or 20 minutes after she receives pain medication.

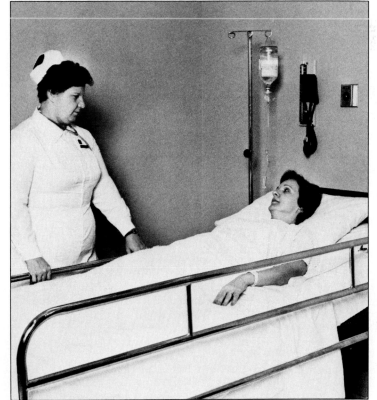

2 If you're certain the patient's ready for ambulation, explain the procedure to her. Stress that ambulation actually promotes healing and improves her body functions. (Chances are, regaining some mobility will boost her spirits, too.) Remember, your patient's cooperation is essential.

Next, obtain slippers with nonskid soles. Also, obtain her bathrobe, if she wishes, or if you plan to help her walk outside her room.

Lower the bed's side rail, as the nurse is doing here. (If your patient has an I.V. line in place, choose the side the I.V. pole is on.) *Caution:* Never leave the patient when the side rail is lowered. Even though she's ready for ambulation, she still needs your support and supervision.

Ongoing care

Ambulating your patient continued

3 Now, lower the bed to its lowest level, so that the patient's feet will touch the floor when she sits on the edge of the bed. This makes standing up as easy as possible for her.

Next, raise the head of the bed to high Fowler's position, to reduce the distance your patient must lift herself when she sits up.

Help your patient move her legs close to the edge of the bed, as shown here. With her legs positioned this way, she'll be able to slide them off the bed easily.

Note: If necessary, help your patient to a sitting position. To do so, stand facing her. Place one foot slightly in front of the other and bend your knees. Place your arms around her, under her arms. Firmly position your hands on her scapulae. Have her place her hands on your shoulders and ease herself to the edge of the bed.

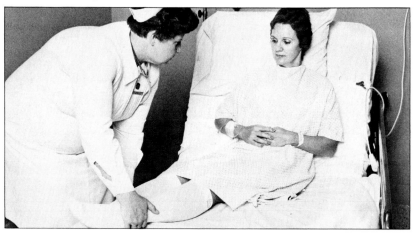

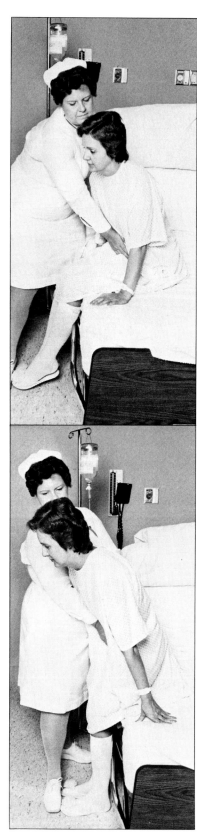

5 If your patient doesn't become dizzy, or if her dizziness is temporary, you may proceed. Put nonskid slippers on her feet. Then, instruct her to grasp the edge of the bed to help support herself. If she has an abdominal incision, splint it for her, as the nurse is doing in the top photo to the left. Then, encourage her to stand up, as shown below.

Note: If your patient's extremely weak, you may have to assist her as follows: Stand facing her and bend your knees. Have her place her hands on your shoulders. Use good body mechanics to help her to a standing position. (If your patient's very heavy, ask a co-worker to help you.)

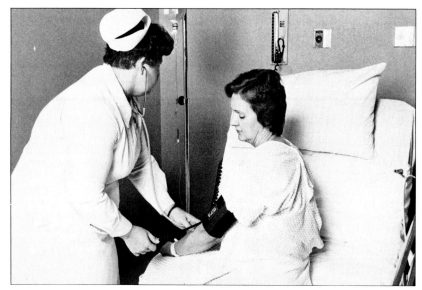

4 Now, help her attain a balanced sitting position. After she's sitting upright, encourage her to take deep breaths. Then, take her blood pressure. Compare it with the blood pressure you recorded earlier. If your patient's experiencing hypotension, slowly lower her back to bed.

Note: Your patient may experience temporary dizziness from postural hypotension. Reassure her that temporary dizziness is normal. If you suspect excessive dizziness (even if she doesn't complain about it) slowly lower her back to bed. Then, document the problem in your nurses' notes and notify the doctor.

6 Then, ask your patient to stand erect. Standing erect will help her maintain balance, strengthen her abdominal muscles, and reduce any muscle strain.

📞 *Nursing tip:* Instruct your patient to look forward, not down. Looking down may make her dizzy.

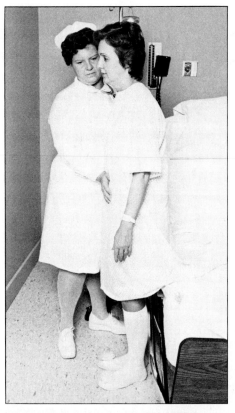

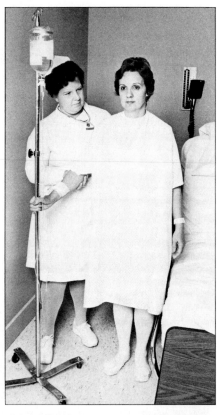

7 If your patient can stand erect, she's ready to walk. To help her do so, stand beside her. Gently grasp her elbow, or allow her to hold your arm. If she has an I.V. line in place, instruct her to push the I.V. pole ahead of her, as shown. Slowly begin walking.

Important: Encourage your patient to steady herself, but not to lean heavily on you. However, be sure to maintain a position which will allow you to support the patient in case she loses her balance.

At first, walk only the distance that seems appropriate for the patient's condition. Gradually increase this distance each time she ambulates. After two or three times, your patient should be able to walk without your direct assistance.

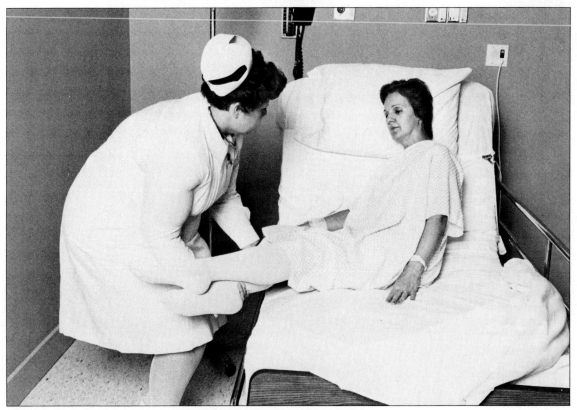

8 After ambulation, return your patient to her bed. Have her resume a sitting position. Then, help her take off her slippers. Help her to lean back against the raised head of the bed, as you lift her legs back into bed. Provide assistance as needed, until she's comfortably positioned in bed. Once again, take her pulse and blood pressure, to detect any changes.

Remember to document the ambulation, including time, distance walked, and patient response (including changes in pulse rate and blood pressure), in your nurses' notes.

Ongoing care

Providing adequate postoperative nutrition

For proper wound healing and rapid convalescence, your patient needs adequate fluids and nutrition after surgery. In the last section, we'll discuss the effects of fluid and electrolyte imbalances. But for now, let's consider postoperative nutrition.

For the first 24 to 48 hours postop, your patient may be unable to eat. Why? Because, depending on the location of the surgical site, peristalsis may be slowed or stopped. Also, a patient may feel nauseated during the first day or so after surgery—possibly as a side effect of the pain medication he's taking. Let your patient resume his normal diet gradually. Remember, the sooner he does so, the quicker his normal gastrointestinal (GI) function will return, because eating stimulates production of digestive juices and promotes intestinal peristalsis. After the immediate postoperative period, you'll assess your patient's GI system at least once each day to determine whether his gastrointestinal function is returning to normal.

If your patient can't eat, he'll probably have a nasogastric (NG) tube in place for elimination of flatus and removal of stomach secretions. While he has the NG tube in place, maintain hydration intravenously (as ordered). If he's extremely weak or debilitated— or if surgery has been extensive—he may even require total parenteral nutrition.

When peristalsis has returned (indicated by auscultation of normal bowel sounds) and the patient feels less nauseated, the doctor may order sips of water or ice chips for him. Can he tolerate the water? If so, the doctor may order a clear liquid diet: tea, fruit juices, clear gelatin, and broth. Your patient should find these bland liquids easy to keep down. But, because they lack high nutritional content, don't continue your patient on this diet for longer than a few days. As soon as he can tolerate the clear liquids well, start him on a soft diet of custard, junket, creamed soups, milk, soft dairy products, and other easily-digested foods, such as stewed chicken and mashed potatoes.

Your patient's goal is to return to a regular diet (or any special diet he may have been on preoperatively) within 3 days after surgery. For optimum recovery, this diet should be high in protein, calories, and minerals, as well as rich in vitamin C (to promote wound healing). If your patient's overweight and prefers to eat fewer calories, provide a high-protein, low-calorie diet. Also, be sure he's receiving enough liquids with it.

Observe your patient's oral intake to see how he tolerates each new stage of his diet. If he's troubled by nausea or gas pains, offer carbonated beverages to help settle his stomach. If the patient's severely nauseated, the doctor may order medication (possibly in suppository form), such as promethazine hydrochloride (Phenergan*) or prochlorperazine maleate (Compazine).

Note: Never force your patient to eat. Doing so may diminish his appetite still further, or stimulate vomiting.

*Available in both the United States and in Canada

Understanding postoperative exercise

As you know, early ambulation helps prevent complications and hastens your patient's recovery from surgery. A patient who's had elective surgery may be able to ambulate within a few hours postoperatively. If he can, he probably won't need a specific exercise program. Some simple feet- and knee-flexing exercises that promote circulation will suffice (see illustrations below).

But, what about a patient who's extremely weak or debilitated, one who's had extensive surgery, or one who develops complications? He may not be able to ambulate shortly after surgery. So, the doctor may order a range-of-motion exercise program for him. By performing range-of-motion exercises, your patient uses his joints to their fullest extent. In addition, he stimulates circulation and promotes muscle tone.

The doctor will choose one of the following three types of range-of-motion programs, depending on your patient's needs:
• active exercises, which the patient performs himself
• active-assistive exercises, which the patient performs with minimal assistance
• passive exercises, which you or another person performs for the patient by moving his limbs.

Depending on your hospital's policy, you will probably collaborate with the patient's doctor and his physical therapist to formulate a specific exercise program. For example, the doctor may instruct a postthoracotomy patient to practice the exercises shown in the self-care aid on the next page. If so, teach the patient to correctly perform them. Then, give him a copy of the aid to take home. (For details on other common range-of-motion exercises, see the NURSING PHOTOBOOKS PROVIDING EARLY MOBILITY and COPING WITH NEUROLOGIC DISORDERS.)

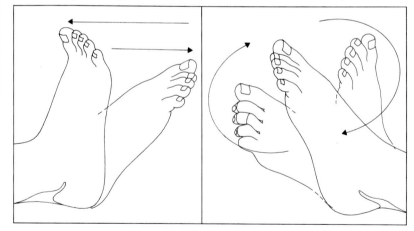

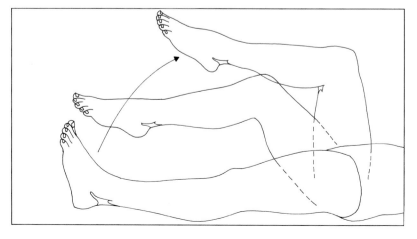

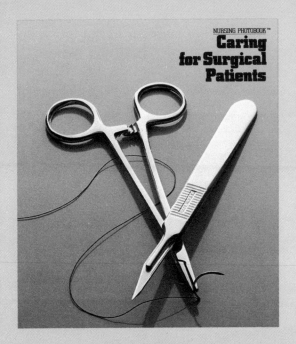

NURSING PHOTOBOOK™
Caring for Surgical Patients

With the help of this PHOTOBOOK, you'll learn to give more competent care for your surgical patient—from the moment he enters the hospital to the day he leaves. You'll find step-by-step instruction on
- preop assessment procedures
- patient teaching
- routine postop care
- wound management
- wound infection control
- and more.

Send for this PHOTOBOOK now and examine it for 10 days...absolutely free.

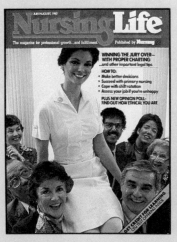

NEW!

FROM THE PUBLISHER OF NURSING84® MAGAZINE.

Mail the postage-paid card at right. ▶

Introduce yourself to the NURSING PHOTOBOOK™ series

…the remarkable breakthrough in nursing education that can change your career. Each book in this unique series contains detailed *Photostories*…and tables, charts, and graphs to help you learn important new procedures. And each handsome PHOTOBOOK offers you • 160 illustrated, fact-filled pages • brilliant, high-contrast, photographs • convenient $9'' \times 10\frac{1}{2}''$ size • durable, hardcover binding • carefully chosen bibliography • complete index. Watch the experts at work showing you how to… administer drugs…teach your patient about his illness and its treatment…minimize trauma… understand doctors' diagnoses…increase patient comfort…and much more. Discover how you can become a better nurse by joining this exciting new series. You can examine each PHOTOBOOK at your liesure…for 10 days *absolutely free!*

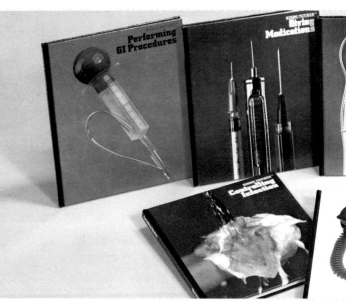

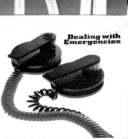

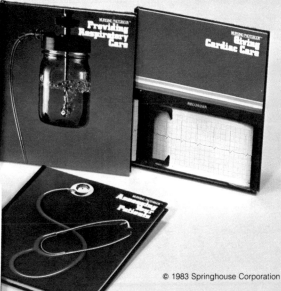

© 1983 Springhouse Corporation

At last! A magazine that helps you with "the other side" of nursing. The things they didn't (and couldn't) teach you in nursing school.

NursingLife tells you how to be a better nurse…how to find greater fulfillment in your career…how to grow on the job.

It's all about the skills today's nurses need to round out their professional lives.

Become a subscriber to this exciting new magazine. Just tear off and mail this card today. There's no need to send money now. This is a no-obligation, free trial offer!

If order card is missing, send your order to:

Nursing Life®

P.O. Box 1961
One Health Care Circle
Marion, Ohio 43305

Self-care

How to strengthen your muscles after a thoracotomy

1 Dear Patient:
The nurse has shown you exercises that will strengthen the arm, shoulder, and chest muscles affected by your surgery. Perform these exercises with your affected arm at least five times each day, and repeat each exercise at least three times.

For your first exercise, lift your shoulders. Hunch your shoulders forward, as shown here, and then pull them back as far as possible.

4 Then, bend your arm at your elbow, so the hand on your affected side rests on your abdomen. Use your opposite hand to grasp your wrist. Raise your arm off your abdomen and bring it directly over the top of your head, inhaling as you do so. Then, as you exhale, lower your arm.

2 Next, raise your elbow, bringing it as close to your ear as possible. Then, extend your arm straight out at shoulder level.

5 Place your arm at your side, with your palm facing forward. Then, raise your arm to the side, bending it over the top of your head. Keep your palm facing forward. Again, inhale as you raise your arm and exhale as you lower it.

3 Now, place your hands on the small of your back. Try to push your elbows and your shoulder blades toward one another.

6 Finally, hold your arm out to your side at shoulder level, with your elbow bent as shown here. Move your forearm straight up and then move it straight down.
Remember: Try to use your affected arm in as many of your daily activities as possible.

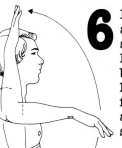

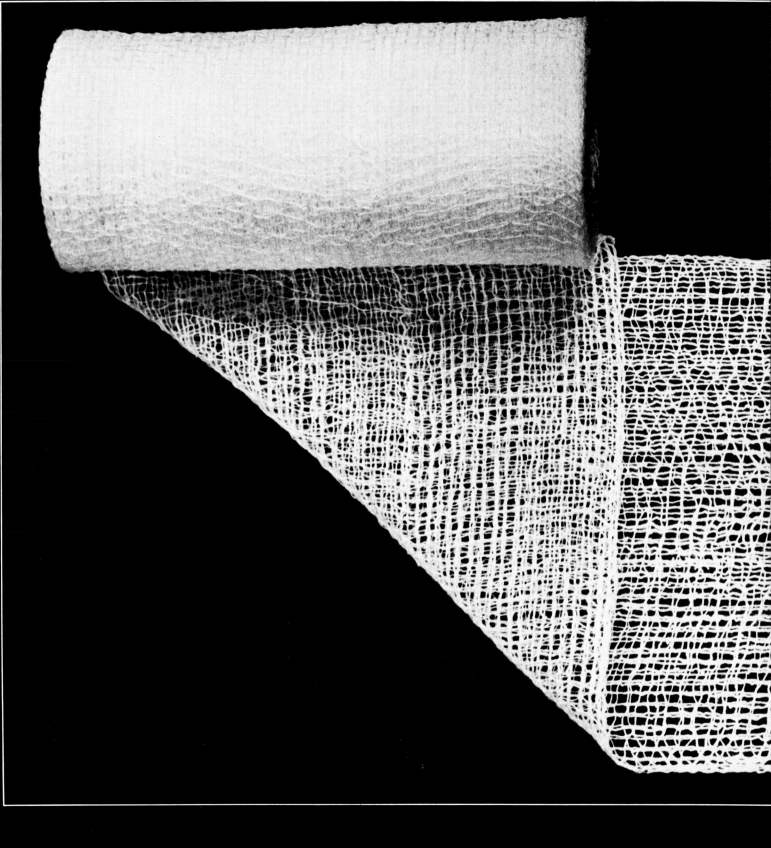

Performing Special Procedures

Wound care
Draining wounds

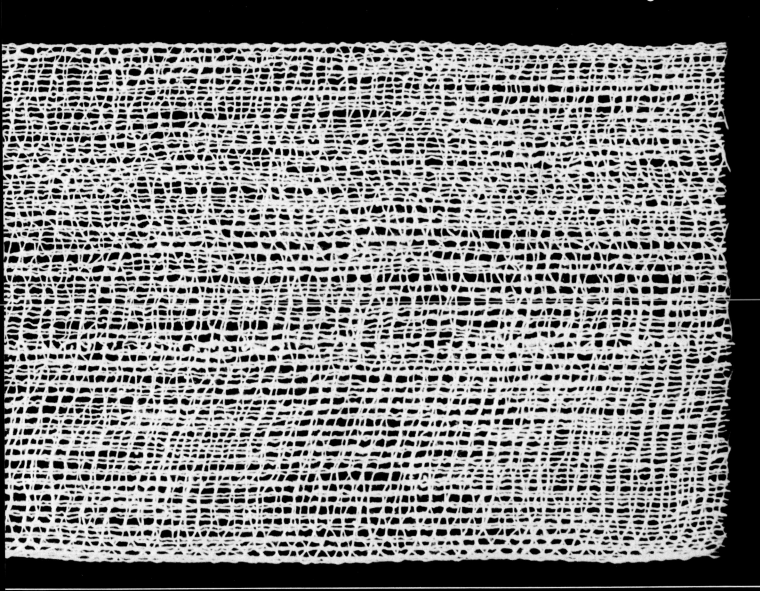

Wound care

Sixty-two-year-old Elena Gomez has returned to your unit after abdominal surgery. Although her family is more relaxed now that the surgery's over, you're less so, because you know that a complex healing process has just begun.

How much do you understand about surgical wounds? For example, do you know how to assess a wound immediately after surgery? Or what to do when a dressing becomes soiled—and the doctor's left orders not to change it?

In the next few pages, you'll find the answers. In addition, we'll take you step-by-step through a complete dressing change and show you how to apply a wet-to-dry dressing. Study this section carefully.

Assessing a surgical wound

Make routine, systematic wound assessment an important part of your postoperative nursing care. To do this, establish a data baseline by frequently inspecting your patient's wound, especially during the first 24 hours after surgery. By doing so, you can quickly identify and assess changes as soon as they occur.

As you assess your patient's wound, ask yourself these questions:
• Is the skin surrounding the wound red, or warm to the touch? If so, document your findings. Note the extent of redness in centimeters, and indicate if you feel warmth.
• What is the proximity of the wound's edges to one another? Document in centimeters any changes that occur.
• What is the condition of the wound's sutures or staples? Have they pulled out or are they tearing the patient's skin? If so, notify the doctor.
• Is the wound bleeding? If so, how much and how often?

Changing your patient's dressing

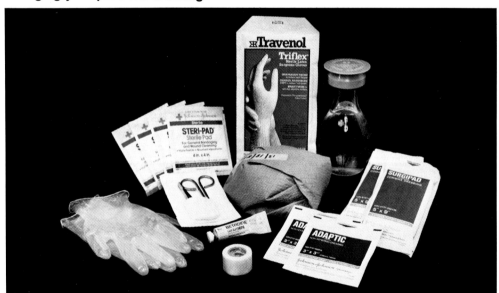

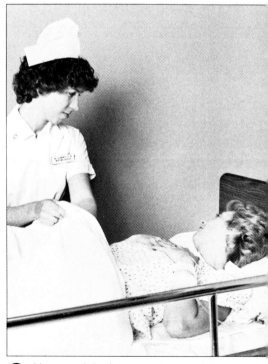

1 *Consider the following situation: Krystal Harper, a 37-year-old pianist, returns to your unit after a hysterectomy. The doctor's ordered Ms. Harper's dressing changed every 12 hours, or as needed. He's also ordered that the wound be cleansed with sterile water, and povidone-iodine ointment applied with each dressing change. Do you know how to proceed? If you're unsure, follow these steps:*

First, prepare for the procedure by gathering the following sterile equipment: nonadhering dressings, 4"x4" gauze pads, a pair of gloves, basin, Surgipads™, and a dress-ing set containing scissors and forceps.

You'll also need: a container of sterile water, povidone-iodine ointment, one pair of non-sterile gloves, nonallergenic tape, and a bed-saver pad and a plastic bag for dressing disposal (not shown).

Note: You may use sterile water, sterile normal saline solution, or povidone-iodine solution to cleanse the wound (as ordered). But, don't use hydrogen peroxide solution with povidone-iodine, because it forms a crust over the wound.

Clear and clean the overbed table. Wash your hands and dry them with a paper towel.

2 Now, explain the procedure and its purpose to Ms. Harper. Also take this opportunity to teach her as much as possible about proper wound care.

Then, expose Ms. Harper's dressing. Tuck a bed-saver pad under her side in the area of the wound. Provide drapes to keep her warm and protect her privacy. Put the opened plastic bag nearby.

Document the number and type of dressings applied, and their size, along with the time of each dressing change or reinforcement.
• Is the wound draining? If so, document the amount, color, odor, and consistency of the drainage. (To learn how to evaluate wound drainage, see the chart on page 112.)
• Does the patient respond normally to a sensory stimulus, such as touch, distal to the wound? Assess his response for any possible loss of sensation.
  To complete your wound assessment, you'll need to evaluate your patient's vital signs. In addition, assess his mental alertness, and the location and intensity of any pain he feels. Note whether movement, position changes, or any other factors aggravate his pain.
  Document all your observations *in detail* in your nurses' notes. And remember, if a significant change occurs, notify the doctor immediately.

Changing the dressing: Some tips

Improperly stored, applied, or discarded dressings or equipment can be a potential infection source. Always follow strict aseptic technique when changing your patient's dressings. Follow these guidelines closely:
• Check sterile equipment for holes, tears, or punctures in the packaging before opening.
• Check the expiration dates on all supplies and equipment.
• Wash your hands with soap or an antimicrobial cleansing agent and dry them with a paper towel before and after all dressing changes. In some cases, you'll need to wash your hands during the dressing change, too.
• Put on gloves before touching heavily-soiled dressings.
• Discard all soiled dressings and disposable equipment in a plastic bag. Then, discard the bag, following your hospital's infection control standards.
• Whenever possible, use single-use bottles of sterile normal saline solution, medicated irrigating solution, and sterile water.
• If you don't have single-use bottles of these solutions, label each bottle with your patient's name, the date, and time. Keep these bottles at your patient's bedside and use them for him only. Discard each bottle within 8 hours of opening, even if it's not empty.
• Whenever possible, use single-use containers or packages of antimicrobial solution and ointment.
• Document all procedures in your nurses' notes.

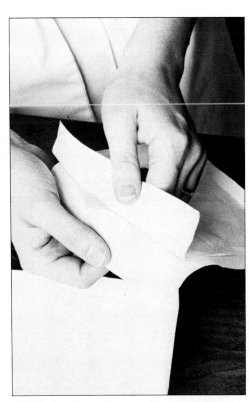

3 Following strict aseptic technique, open the packages of sterile 4″x4″ gauze pads. Leaving the pads in their open wrappers, place them on the overbed table. Follow this procedure with the nonadhering dressings, Surgipads, scissors, and forceps.

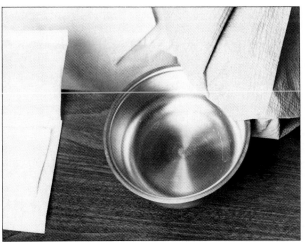

4 Maintaining sterility, remove the wrapper from the basin. Place the basin on the overbed table, taking care not to contaminate its inside.

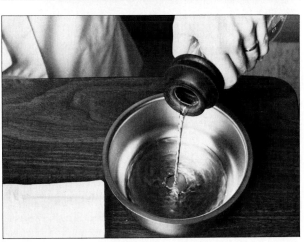

5 Then, remove the cap from the sterile water container. Pour about 50 ml of water into the basin. To avoid contamination, take care not to touch the bottle to the basin, or to splash water on the sterile field.
  Touching only the outside of the bottle cap, replace the cap on the water container. Place the bottle on the bedside table.

Wound care

Changing your patient's dressing continued

6 Now you're ready to remove the tape from Ms. Harper's dressing. To do this, put on the nonsterile gloves. Applying gentle tension to her skin with one hand, pull the tape toward the wound with your other hand, as shown here.

Note: Always use short, quick pulls to minimize suture strain and patient discomfort.

Place the soiled tape in the plastic bag.

Gently remove the soiled dressings one at a time, folding them together so they don't contaminate your gloves. *Caution:* Never pull on a dressing. Doing so may disturb sutures or newly-formed tissue.

💨 *Nursing tip:* Suppose you have difficulty removing a dressing. Try moistening the area with sterile water or normal saline solution.

Place the soiled dressings in the plastic bag. Remove your gloves and place them in the plastic bag, too. Wash your hands.

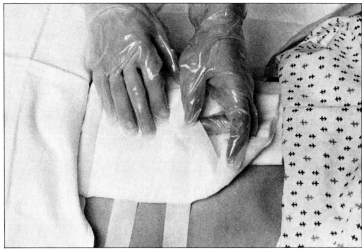

8 Now, dip the folded gauze pad into the sterile water. Take care to point the forceps and gauze pad downward, so the excess water drips into the basin.

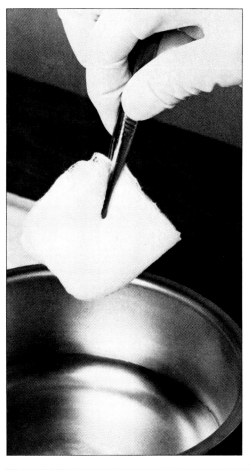

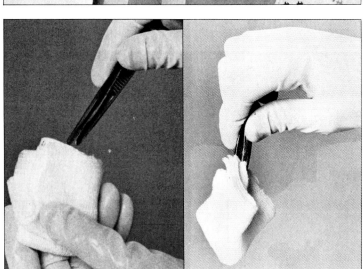

7 Put on your sterile gloves, following the procedure shown on page 48. Carefully inspect your patient's wound for any discharge or redness. If you see any, notify the doctor after you complete the dressing change.

Then, fold a 4"x4" gauze pad into quarters and grasp it with the forceps, as shown at left. Make sure the folded edge faces outward, as shown at right.

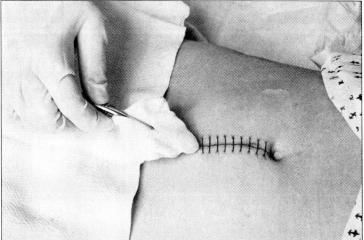

9 Starting at the top of the incision, gently wipe from top to bottom in one motion.

Then, discard the gauze pad in the plastic bag. To avoid contamination, don't touch the bag with the forceps. Repeat this procedure, wiping in the same direction each time. Always move from the least-contaminated area to the most-contaminated area. Using a clean gauze pad with each wiping motion, continue the procedure until you've cleansed the entire wound.

10 Using a 4″x4″ gauze pad, pat the area dry, as shown in this photo. Discard all used gauze pads in the plastic bag.

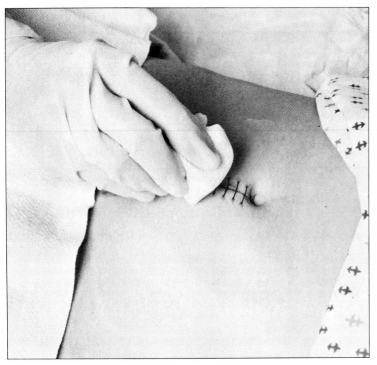

11 Now, using only your nondominant hand, remove the cap from the tube of povidone-iodine ointment. Remember, this hand is no longer sterile.

Using the same hand, squeeze a small amount of ointment onto a 4″x4″ gauze pad and discard the pad. Doing so ensures ointment sterility.

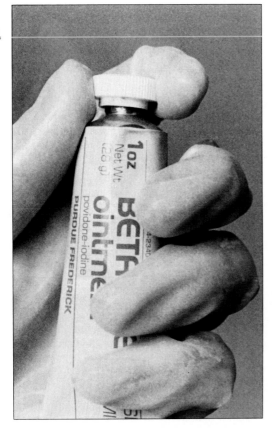

12 Squeeze ointment over your patient's entire wound from top to bottom, as the nurse is doing here. Take care not to touch her wound with the top of the ointment tube. And remember, use this tube *only* for Ms. Harper.

Using your nondominant hand, recap the ointment and put it aside. Be sure to use only your dominant hand to apply the sterile dressings, since your nondominant hand is no longer sterile.

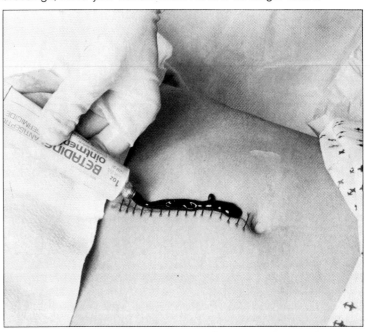

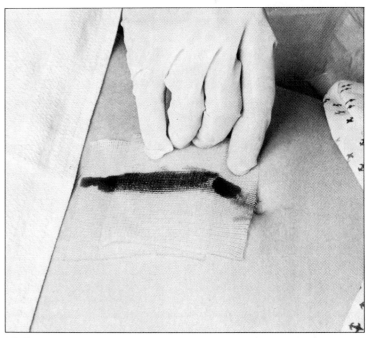

13 To prevent the primary dressing from sticking to the wound, place the nonadhering dressing over the wound. Use two nonadhering dressings if necessary to cover the entire wound, as shown. Check to be sure the wound's completely covered.

Wound care

Changing your patient's dressing continued

14 To apply the primary dressing, remove a 4"x4" gauze pad from its open wrapper. Place the pad over the nonadhering dressings. Repeat this procedure until you've covered the nonadhering dressings.

Remember, the primary dressing will help absorb drainage from the wound surface.

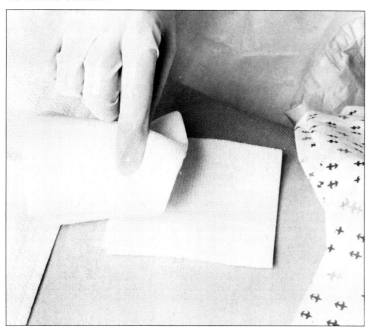

16 Place two parallel strips of tape across the dressing, as the nurse is doing here. Attach the center of each tape strip to the middle of the dressing.

Then, applying gentle pressure, smooth both sides of the tape outward toward the ends. This distributes tension away from the wound.

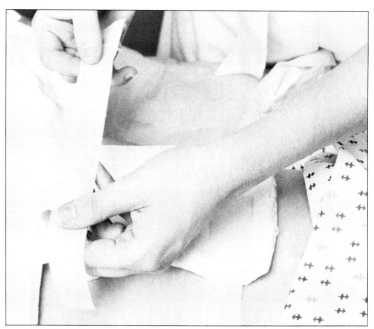

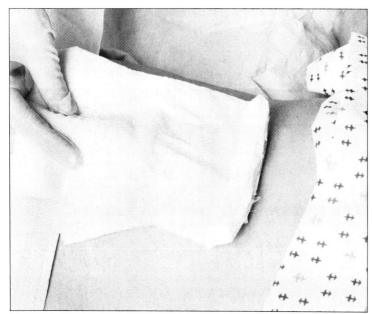

15 Now, you're ready to apply the secondary dressing, which will act as a drainage reservoir. To proceed, place a Surgipad directly over the gauze pads, as shown.(If necessary to cover the wound, apply a second Surgipad.)

🔖 *Nursing tip:* Fold the Surgipad so the thickest part is over the wound's dependent side; drainage will flow in that direction.

Remove your gloves, and discard them in the plastic bag.

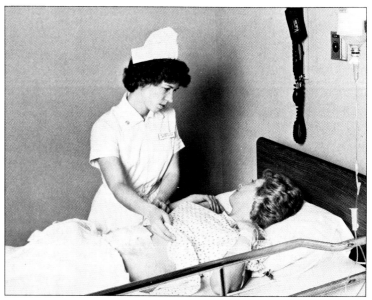

17 Adjust your patient's linens, and make her comfortable. Then, discard all disposable instruments and supplies in the plastic bag. Close the bag with a fastener and discard it according to your hospital's infection control standards. Never leave it in the patient's room. Wash your hands.

Finally, document the procedure in your nurses' notes, including the appearance of the wound and surrounding skin, and the amount, color, odor, and consistency of drainage.

Reinforcing the dressing

1 *Walter Sedgwick, a 28-year-old apprentice electrician, arrives in your unit from the recovery room. Three hours ago, Mr. Sedgwick had a partial nephrectomy. The doctor has left orders that he'll make the initial dressing change 24 hours postop. He's also warned you to expect copious drainage. When you examine the dressing, you see that the edges are saturated with drainage. Since the doctor doesn't want you to change the dressing, you'll need to reinforce it. Here's how:*

Begin by reassuring Mr. Sedgwick. Explain the procedure as you perform it, even if he seems groggy from the anesthetic.

Then, gather the equipment you'll need: several Surgipads and nonallergenic tape. In case the reinforced dressing becomes saturated, you'll also need a plastic bag and nonsterile gloves.

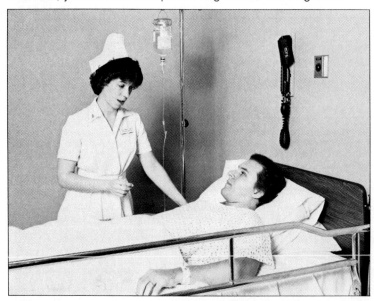

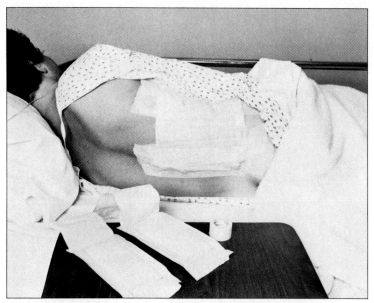

2 Wash your hands and dry them with a paper towel. Then, open the Surgipad wrappers. Leaving the Surgipads in their wrappers, place them on the bedside table.

3 Taking care to touch only the outside of the pads, place them over the wet dressing's edges, as the nurse is doing here. Repeat this procedure until you've covered the entire saturated area. Then, securely tape the pads in place.

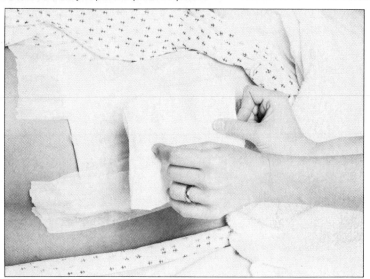

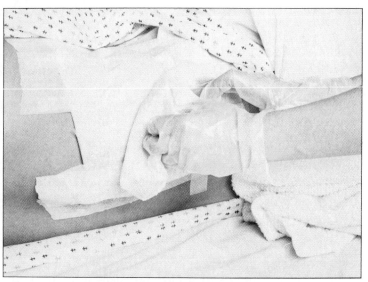

4 Suppose, after a few hours, the dressing's reinforced section becomes saturated. Put on a pair of nonsterile gloves. Then, remove the Surgipads you used to reinforce the original dressing, as the nurse is doing here. Discard the soiled Surgipads in a plastic bag. Then, following the guidelines in step 3, cover the primary dressing with the clean Surgipads, and tape them in place. Dispose of the plastic bag.

Closely monitor the surgical site for continued drainage. Encircle wet areas, so you can evaluate any changes. If the dressing again becomes saturated, notify the doctor.

Note: When caring for a surgical patient in a nursing unit, don't reinforce his dressing more than two times without notifying the doctor.

Finally, document the procedure in your nurses' notes. Include the date and time, drainage consistency, color, and odor.

Wound care

Applying a wet-to-dry dressing

1 *If your patient has an open surgical wound, the doctor may order a wet-to-dry dressing to prevent a suspected infection from developing. To apply such a dressing, you'll moisten sterile gauze pads with antimicrobial solution, as ordered by the doctor, and place the pads into the wound. As the wet dressing dries, any necrotic tissue on the wound's surface adheres to it. When you remove the dressing, you also remove the necrotic tissue.*

This helps debride the wound and stimulate healing. To apply a wet-to-dry dressing, read this photostory.

First, obtain this equipment: a pair of sterile gloves, a pair of nonsterile gloves, several 4"x4" gauze pads, a single-use bottle of povidone-iodine solution (Betadine*), a roll of sterile gauze, nonallergenic tape, and a bed-saver pad and plastic trash bag (not shown).

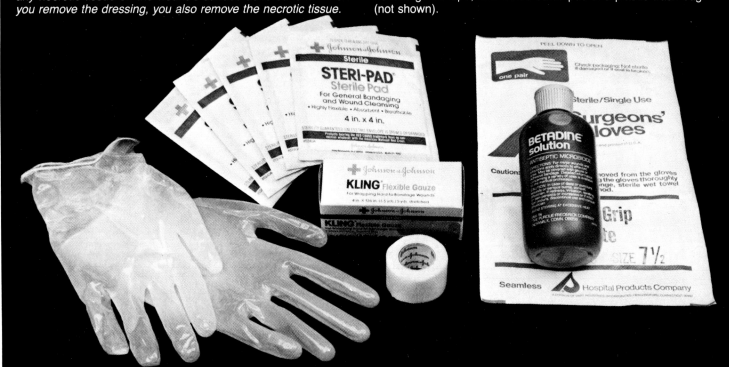

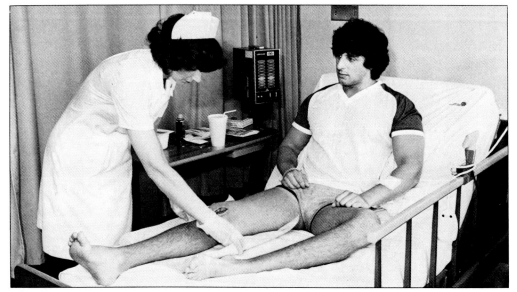

2 Put on your nonsterile gloves, and remove the patient's soiled dressing. (See page 106.) Inspect the wound. Then, explain the procedure to the patient. If you haven't done so already, place a bed-saver pad under the patient's wound.

Remove your nonsterile gloves and dispose of them properly. Wash and dry your hands.

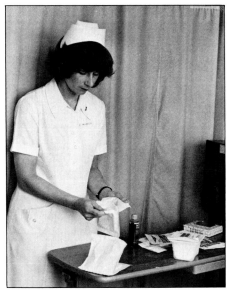

3 Open several 4"x4" gauze pads, using aseptic technique. To prevent contamination, leave the pads on their sterile wrappers.

*Available in both the United States and in Canada

4 Take the bottle of povidone-iodine solution and squirt the solution over the pad, as shown. Make sure you don't contaminate the pad by touching it with the bottle's top.

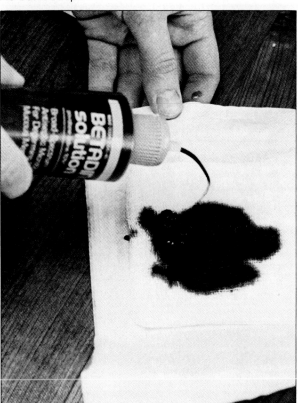

6 Take another moistened gauze pad and gently push it into the wound, as the nurse is about to do in this photo. Repeat this procedure until you've completely filled the wound. Then, lay one or two moistened pads over the wound.

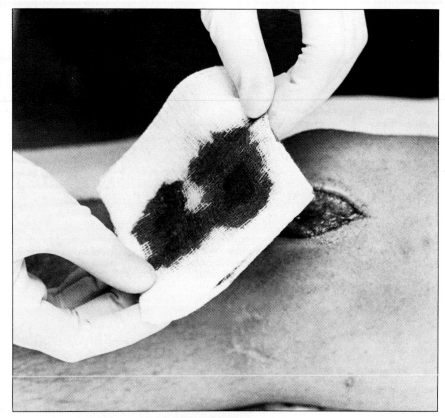

5 Now, put on sterile gloves. Take the moistened pad and squeeze out excess solution, if necessary. Then, cleanse the wound with the pad, maintaining sterile technique. Wipe the wound from the inside, working in one direction from the middle of the wound to its edge. Don't use the same pad more than once. And don't touch the wound with your gloves.

Repeat this procedure until the wound is cleansed. Dispose of the soiled pads properly.

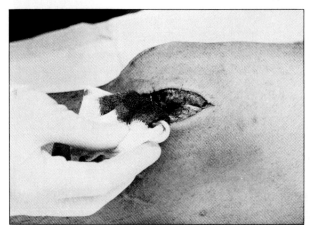

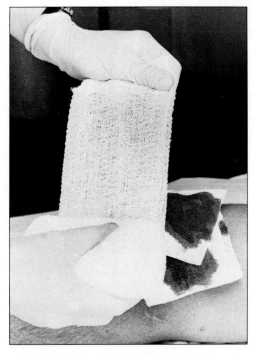

7 Secure the wet-to-dry dressing by wrapping gauze around the dressing, as the nurse is doing here. Remove your gloves, and dispose of them in the plastic bag. Secure the dressing with nonallergenic tape. *Note:* If the wound is on another area of the patient's body (such as his abdomen), cover the wet-to-dry dressing with dry pads, and secure the entire dressing with Montgomery straps.

Remove your gloves and dispose of them in the plastic bag. Tape the dressing with nonallergenic tape. Then, dispose of soiled equipment according to your hospital's infection control standards. Wash and dry your hands.

Document the procedure in your nurses' notes. Also, document the appearance of the wound and surrounding skin.

Draining wounds

If you're like most nurses, you dread caring for a patient with a draining surgical wound. Why? Because, depending on the size of the wound and the type of drainage, wound and skin care can present enormous challenges for you.

In the following pages, we'll help you provide the very best care for a patient with a draining wound. For example, we'll show you how to:
• change a dressing around a drain.
• make and apply Montgomery straps.

• use a surgical wound evacuator.
• apply a skin barrier around a wound or a drain.
• apply a disposable pouch to a draining wound.
     Sound helpful? Read on.

Nurses' guide to abdominal wound drainage

After most types of abdominal surgery, you expect to see wound drainage. But how *much* drainage is normal, and what should it look like?

Take a look at this chart. It provides a guide to the amount and appearance of drainage you can expect after some common abdominal surgeries.

Procedure	Day of surgery	1st day postop	2nd, 3rd day postop	4th day to discharge
Abdominal-perineal resection	• profuse • serosanguineous	• moderate • serosanguineous	• moderate • serous	• minimal • serous
Appendectomy (simple)	• minimal • serous (brownish)	• minimal • serous	• none	• none
Appendectomy (with rupture)	• moderate • purulent, brownish-green	• moderate • purulent	• minimal • serous	• minimal • serous
Cholecystectomy (without T tube to bile bag)	• moderate to profuse • sanguineous with bile	• moderate • bile (brown)	• moderate • brown, serous	• minimal • serous
Colectomy	• moderate • serosanguineous	• minimal • serous	• minimal • serous	• minimal • serous
Cystectomy	• moderate • serosanguineous	• minimal • serous	• minimal • serous	• minimal • serous
Gastrectomy	• moderate • serosanguineous	• moderate • serosanguineous	• minimal • serous	• minimal • serous
Hysterectomy (abdominal)	• minimal • serous	• minimal • serous	• none	• none
Inguinal herniorrhaphy	• minimal • serous	• minimal • serous	• none	• none
Nephrectomy, nephroureterectomy	• moderate • sanguineous	• moderate • serosanguineous	• minimal • serous	• minimal • serous
Pyelolithotomy	• profuse • serosanguineous (urine)	• profuse • serous (urine)	• profuse • urine	• moderate to minimal • urine
Ovarian cystectomy	• minimal • serous	• minimal • serous	• minimal • serous	• none
Small bowel resection	• moderate • serosanguineous	• moderate • serosanguineous	• minimal • serous	• minimal • serous
Splenectomy	• moderate • sanguineous	• moderate • serosanguineous	• minimal • serous	• minimal • serous

Learning about drains

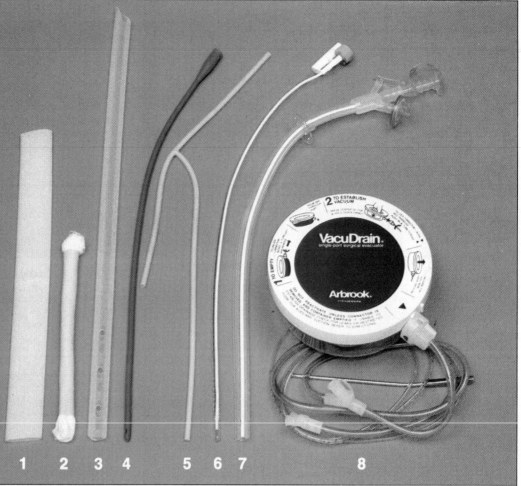

How familiar are you with wound drains? As you probably know, the doctor may insert a drain into—or close to—a surgical wound if he expects large amounts of drainage. How does the doctor select a drain for your patient's wound? That depends on the wound's location, size, and type; the amount of drainage expected; and the equipment available.

Once the drain's inserted, the surgeon may pin or clip the outer end to keep it from slipping into the wound. As the patient's recovery progresses, the doctor periodically will slightly withdraw the drain, to permit healing from within.

The chart that follows will show you several different types of drains.

Note: If your patient's had thoracic surgery, see the NURSING PHOTOBOOK PROVIDING RESPIRATORY CARE for details on chest drainage tubes.

Gravity drains

1. Penrose
Description: Single-lumen, soft latex rubber tube. May have X-ray opaque stripe for placement verification. Can be sutured in place. Available in sizes ranging from ¼" to 1" (0.6 to 2.5 cm) in diameter and 12" to 36" (30 to 91 cm) in length.
Indication: For a patient with a moderately-sized, uncomplicated draining wound.

2. Cigarette
Description: Single-lumen, soft latex rubber tube containing gauze. May have X-ray opaque stripe for placement verification. Can be sutured in place. Available in a variety of sizes.
Indication: For a patient with a moderately-sized, uncomplicated draining wound. This drain prevents the need for suctioning by using gauze to draw up drainage by capillary action.

3. Axion™ mediastinal silicone catheter
Description: Sterile, silicone catheter ¾" (1.9 cm) in diameter. Available in a variety of lengths. Is nontoxic and nonpyrogenic. Can be sutured in place.
Indication: For a patient with a large, draining abdominal or mediastinal wound. May also be attached to suction to evacuate the wound. May be cut if necessary, and drainage bag applied. Large size of catheter permits easy irrigation, if necessary.

4. Davol® rubber suction catheter (Red Robinson tube)
Description: Soft, flexible red rubber or plastic tube or catheter. Available in a variety of sizes. Can be sutured in place.
Indication: For a patient with an uncomplicated, moderately-sized draining wound. May also be attached to low suction to evacuate the wound.

5. T tube
Description: Silicone catheter with a stem and perforated crossbar. Available in a variety of sizes.
Indication: For a patient requiring common bile duct drainage.

Sump drains

6. Double-lumen (Shirley®)
Description: Double-lumen silicone or plastic tube with ingress portion smaller than egress. This drain uses air entering through ingress portion to help draw drainage into the egress portion for removal. May come with X-ray opaque stripe for placement verification. Available in a variety of sizes. Can be sutured in place.
Indication: For a patient with a large abdominal wound, an infected wound, or a secondary infection in another area. This product keeps drainage or adjacent tissue from sealing off egress lumen. It also prevents suction damage to delicate internal tissues.

7. Triple-lumen (Davol® Abramson)
Description: Triple-lumen, silicone or plastic tube with large center lumen for drainage removal. Smaller size lumens allow filtered air, medication, or irrigation solution to reach wound. May have X-ray opaque stripe for placement verification. Available in a variety of sizes. Can be sutured in place.
Indication: For a patient with a large draining abdominal wound or infection.

Surgical evacuators

8. VacuDrain™, Vac-U-Care™, Hemovac™
Description: Single-lumen silicone tube attached to evacuator unit. Evacuator unit allows you to measure drainage, then empty it while providing constant suction. Some units also prevent reflux of drainage. To allow ambulation, pin drain to patient's gown below wound.
Indication: For an ambulatory patient with a large draining wound.

Draining wounds

Applying a dressing around a drain

1 *Suppose Frances Mills just had a cholecystectomy, and the doctor inserted a T tube to allow for drainage. You have to change the dressing around the drain. Do you know how?*

First, gather the necessary sterile equipment: scissors, 4"x4" gauze pads, gloves, and a Surgipad. You'll also need nonallergenic tape (or Montgomery straps), a plastic bag to dispose of soiled equipment, and a bed-saver pad. If necessary, also obtain a skin barrier, such as Stomahesive®.

Note: Some hospitals have 4"x4" gauze pads that are already cut. Use them if they're available.

Position the patient so the wound is accessible. Try to drape the patient to maintain her privacy. Explain the procedure and why it's needed.

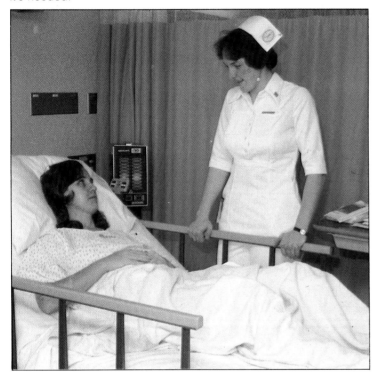

2 Remove your patient's soiled dressing. (If the dressing is heavily soiled, wear non-sterile gloves while removing it.) Then, wash and dry your hands.

Note: If the doctor orders, cleanse the wound (using aseptic technique) before you apply a new dressing.

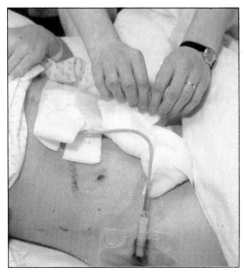

3 Closely inspect the skin around your patient's drain. If you notice any signs of skin irritation, apply a skin barrier such as Stomahesive to protect her skin from further irritation.

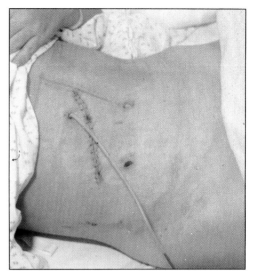

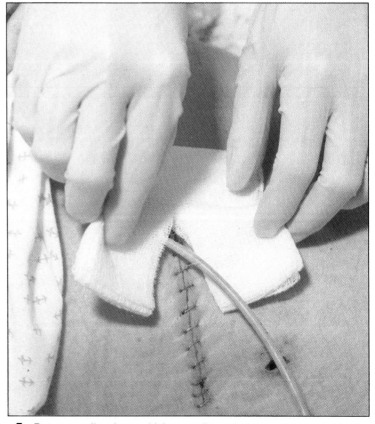

4 Put on sterile gloves. Using sterile technique, pick up a 4"x4" gauze pad with your nondominant hand. Take the scissors in your dominant hand and cut halfway through the pad.

☎ *Nursing tip:* The pad may fit better around a large drain if you snip a small V into the pad at the end of the cut. Cut another 4"x4" pad, following the same procedure.

Now, take each 4"x4" gauze pad and place it snugly around your patient's drain. Make sure the cut portions of the pads overlap. Apply additional 4"x4" pads to cover the wound, if necessary.

5 Remove your gloves and discard them in the plastic bag. Then, unwrap the Surgipad, if you haven't already done so. Place it over the small gauze pads, without touching the Surgipad's underside with your fingers.

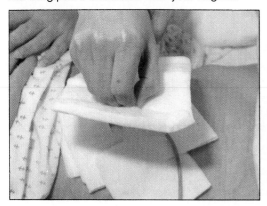

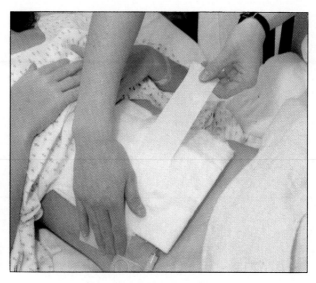

6 Tape the entire dressing into place with nonallergenic tape. Or, secure the dressing with Montgomery straps, as shown in the next photostory.

Finally, place all disposable equipment in the plastic bag. Fasten the bag, and dispose of it according to your hospital's infection control standards. Wash and dry your hands.

Document the procedure and your observations in your nurses' notes. Include the appearance of the wound and skin around the drain, and the amount and color of drainage.

How to make Montgomery straps

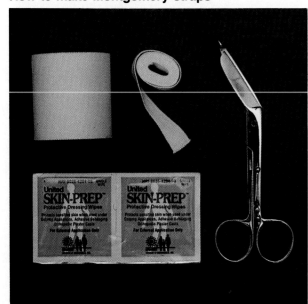

1 *If your patient has a draining wound, he may need frequent dressing changes. To make dressing changes as comfortable as possible for the patient, you'll probably secure his dressings with Montgomery straps. Unless they become wet or soiled, you needn't remove these straps during subsequent dressing changes. As a result, you eliminate the skin trauma and discomfort associated with frequent tape removal.*

If your hospital doesn't carry commercially-made Montgomery straps, you can make your own. We'll show you how to make and apply them in this photostory.

First, obtain 2" nonallergenic tape, scissors, Skin-Prep™, and twill tape.

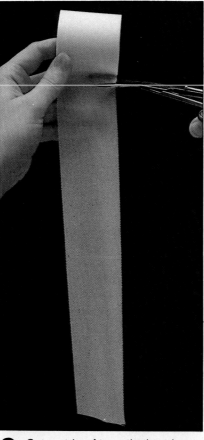

2 Cut a strip of tape that's at least 4" (10.2 cm) longer than the length needed to secure the dressing.

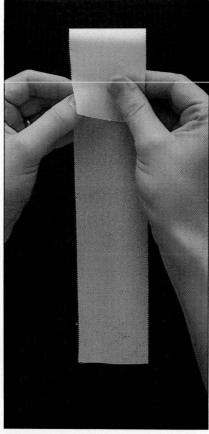

3 Fold one end of the tape back onto itself (sticky sides together) so you have a 2" (5.1 cm) tab.

Draining wounds

How to make Montgomery straps continued

4 Cut a small hole in the folded tab's center, close to its top edge. Make as many pairs of straps as you'll need to snugly secure the dressing. (In this photostory, we'll show two pairs.)

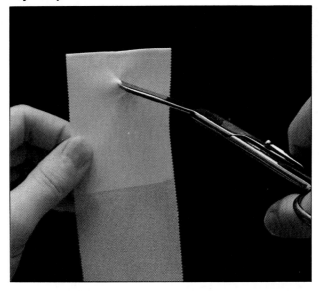

5 To protect the patient's skin, apply Skin-Prep beside his dressing, over the areas where you'll apply the straps. Then, beginning near the dressing, tape one pair of straps over the Skin-Prep. Place part of the folded tab on the dressing, and part over the Skin-Prep.

Now, cut a piece of twill tape that's long enough to double through the holes in both tabs. Then, run the tape through both tabs, as shown.

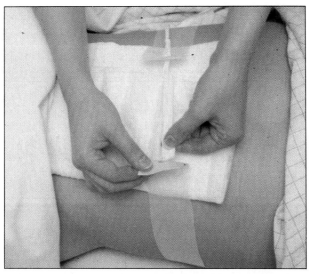

6 Secure the dressing by tying the ends of the tape together, as the nurse is doing here.

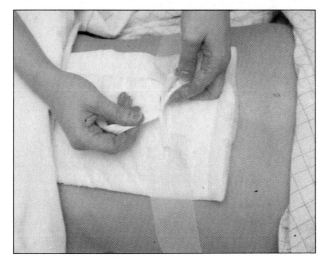

7 Repeat the procedure to apply and secure the other pair of straps.

Nursing tip: If you prefer, use gauze ties instead of twill tape to tie the straps.

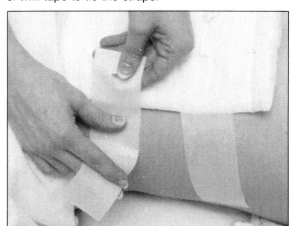

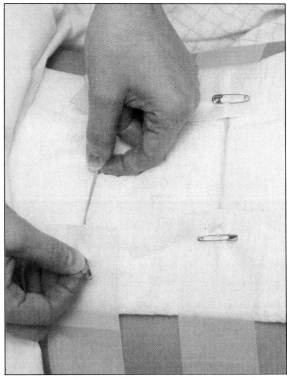

8 As an alternative, secure the straps this way: Slip a rubber band over two open safety pins, and close the pins. Then, insert a closed safety pin in each tab's hole (see the pair of straps on the right). To open the strap, slip the safety pin through the hole of one tab, as the nurse is doing here.

Remember to check the condition of the Montgomery straps when changing the patient's dressing. If the straps are soiled or wet, change them, too.

After you've finished, document the procedure and your observations in your nurses' notes.

Securing a tube with tape

1 *If your patient has a drainage tube in or near his surgical wound to facilitate drainage, you may have to secure the tube with nonallergenic tape. Follow the steps in this photostory to learn the proper procedure.*

First, obtain nonallergenic tape that's 2″ (5.1 cm) wide. Cut a piece long enough to adequately secure the tube. Then, make two lengthwise cuts to the middle of the tape, as shown here. Doing so divides it into thirds.

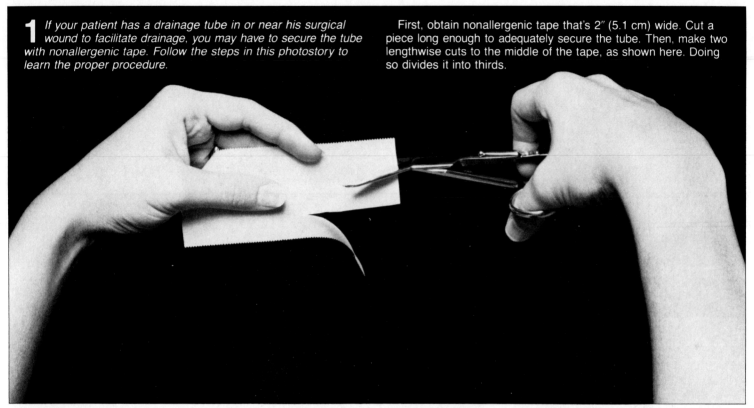

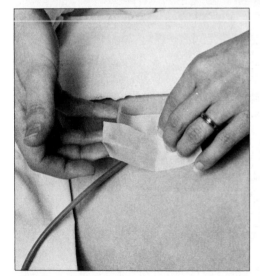

2 Before you begin, apply a skin barrier such as Skin-Prep to protect your patient's skin. Then, place the uncut portion of tape over the Skin-Prep. (If the drain's inserted in the incision, place the tape perpendicular to the incision.) The end of the uncut portion should be next to the tube, as shown. Smooth the uncut portion over the patient's protected skin, starting near the tube and moving away from it.

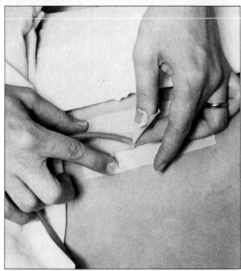

3 Now, turn your attention to the cut portion of tape. Fasten the two outer strips over the Skin-Prep, starting near the tube and working away from it.

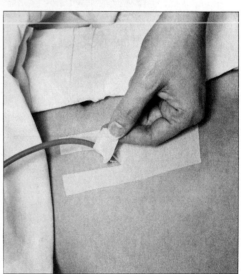

4 Next, take the middle strip and wrap it around the tube in a spiral fashion, as shown here.

Repeat the entire procedure on the opposite side of the tube. Then, if you have to secure the tube further, apply a strip of tape on each side of the tube, perpendicular to the strips already in place (but not directly over an incision).

Document what you've done.

Draining wounds

Caring for a patient with a Vac-U-Care™

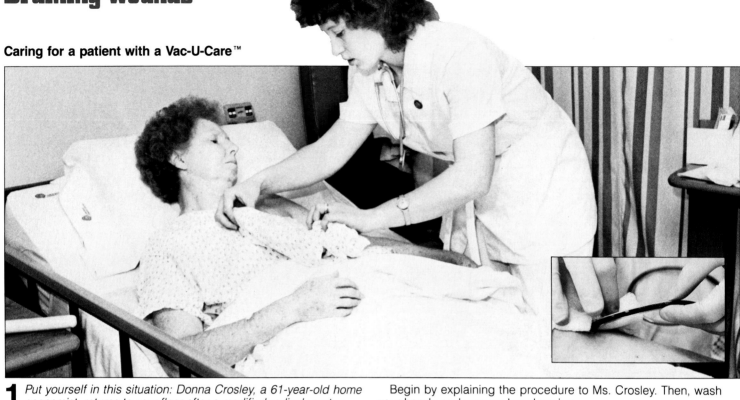

1 *Put yourself in this situation: Donna Crosley, a 61-year-old home economist, returns to your floor after a modified radical mastectomy of her left breast. During surgery, the doctor inserted drainage tubing directly into her wound and connected it to an evacuator container. He's left orders to empty the evacuator container every 8 hours, or as needed. Do you know how? If you're using a Vac-U-Care surgical evacuator, follow these steps:*

Begin by explaining the procedure to Ms. Crosley. Then, wash your hands and expose her dressing.

Inspect her dressing for excessive bleeding or drainage. If you see any, suspect a dislodged or blocked drain. Notify the doctor immediately, and prepare to change the dressing, as ordered.

[Inset] Be sure the perforated portion of the Vac-U-Care tubing remains under your patient's skin to maintain suction.

2 Next, flip open the evacuator container's drainage port.

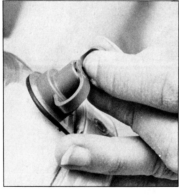

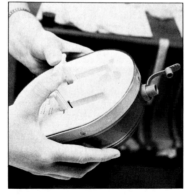

4 To reactivate the vacuum, lift the white handle, as the nurse has done here.

3 Pour the drainage through the port and into a measuring container, as shown in this photo.

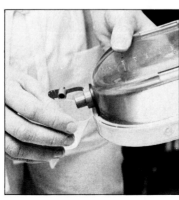

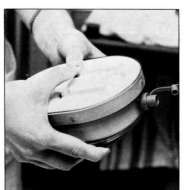

5 Then, push the handle back into the Vac-U-Care unit, as shown in this photo. Close the drainage port.

Measure and discard the drainage, according to infection control standards. Properly discard the container (if it's disposable), and replace it with a new one. Nondisposable containers can be disinfected. Wash your hands.

Document the drainage amount, color, odor, and consistency. Monitor the equipment to make sure it maintains suction.

Choosing drainage pouches

You may think of drainage pouches as being only for patients who have had ostomy surgery. But, when applied with a skin barrier, a pouch can also effectively protect the patient's skin from maceration and excoriation caused by wound drainage. Besides isolating the drainage site from other body sites, the pouch allows you to keep an accurate drainage record. You'll also save time and money by eliminating the need for frequent dressing changes. And, if the wound is infected, the pouch will help prevent the drainage from spreading infection, and control any odor.

Keep in mind that the drainage site may not be at the wound. In such a case, a pouch over the drainage site may eliminate the need for a wound dressing. A drainage pouch is usually more comfortable for your patient than a wound dressing. It also allows you to easily observe and assess the wound.

The chart that follows will acquaint you with several different types of drainage pouches. Always choose a pouch with an opening that's only slightly larger than your patient's drainage site. Position the pouch in the direction of gravitational flow. (Take into consideration any position changes your patient may make.)

Disposable drainage pouches with adhesives

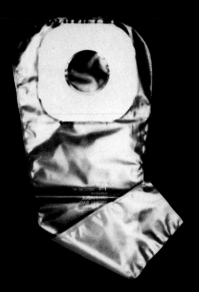

Hollister™ drainable pouch
Clear, odor-proof plastic pouch with preattached adhesive square. Fits drainage sites from 1″ to 3″ (2.5 to 7.6 cm). Some models have belt tabs.

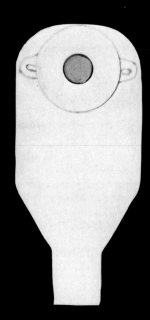

Nu-Hope postop pouch
Opaque, odor-proof plastic pouch with belt tabs. Fits drainage sites from ½″ to 3″ (1.3 to 7.6 cm). Some models have a preattached foam pad.

Disposable drainage pouch with skin barrier

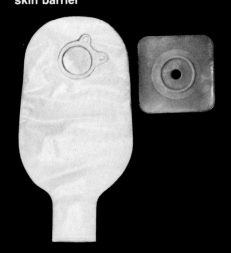

Squibb® Sur-fit® pouch
Transparent or opaque, odor-proof pouch with belt tabs. Snaps to specially-made Stomahesive® with Sur-fit flange. Fits drainage sites from ½″ to 2¾″ (1.3 to 7 cm). This product can be removed and replaced without disturbing skin seal.

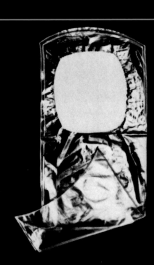

Bongort® pouch
Odor-proof, transparent pouch with adhesive square. Measure and cut adhesive square slightly larger than drainage site. Especially useful for irregularly-shaped drainage sites. Some models come with a cap that's adaptable to an indwelling (Foley) catheter bag.

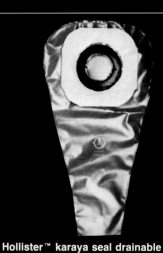

Hollister™ karaya seal drainable stoma pouch
Transparent or opaque, odor-proof plastic pouch with preattached karaya seal. Fits drainage sites from 1″ to 3″ (2.5 to 7.6 cm). Some models may have microporous adhesive or belt tabs. The pouch above features a karaya seal with microporous adhesives. Other models have a karaya seal with belt tabs.

Draining wounds

Applying skin barriers

Whenever you care for a patient with a draining wound, you'll need to protect his skin and monitor its condition, especially around his wound or drain. To ensure skin integrity, apply a skin barrier to this area.

As you probably know, various types of skin barriers are available. When selecting one for your patient, consider product availability, wound location, patient preference, and skin condition. Also consider whether you're going to redress the wound or apply a drainage bag. And, remember, a skin barrier without a precut hole is easier to fit to your patient's wound or drain. Also, keep in mind that some drainage pouches are available with an attached barrier.

After you choose the best product for your patient, learn how to apply it properly. The information that follows will acquaint you with some common types of skin barriers, and their applications.

Before you apply any barriers, follow these guidelines:
• Tell your patient what the barrier will accomplish and how it's applied.
• Use a measuring card or pattern to measure the size of your patient's wound or drain site. *Important:* If you're using Colly Seel®, ReliaSeal™ or Stomahesive®, be sure to cut the opening so that it's no more than 1/8" (0.3 cm) larger than your patient's drain.
• If your patient has a dressing or pouch over his wound or drain, remove it. Place gauze over the wound or drain to absorb any leakage.
📼 *Nursing tip:* A rolled 4"x4" gauze pad or a regular-sized tampon held over your patient's wound or drain will act as a wick to absorb drainage.
• Cleanse the wound area and pat it dry. Be sure to change the gauze over it as often as needed to keep your patient's skin clean.
• After applying any skin barrier, document your observations in your nurses' notes.

To learn how to apply some common skin barriers, examine the following photos.

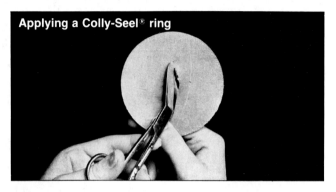

Applying a Colly-Seel® ring

1 Are you using a Colly-Seel ring to protect your patient's skin? If so, cut an opening for your patient's drain which allows only minimal skin exposure.

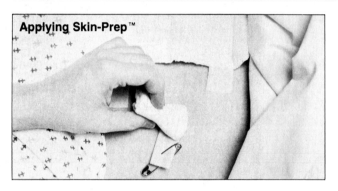

Applying Skin-Prep™

1 As you probably know, Skin-Prep is a solution that you'll brush, wipe, or spray onto the skin around your patient's wound. Here's how:

Begin by covering your patient's wound with a gauze pad to protect it. If you're using a brush applicator, carefully apply a thin layer of the plastic coating around the wound. Let it dry for about 30 seconds.

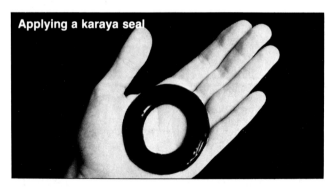

Applying a karaya seal

1 You can get karaya seal in the following forms: as a small or large ring, a sheet, powder, or paste. If you're using a ring, make sure its opening is large enough to fit around the patient's drain.

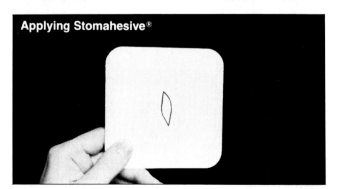

Applying Stomahesive®

1 Applying Stomahesive to your patient's wound? If you're using a Stomahesive sheet, trace your patient's wound size on the Stomahesive backing.

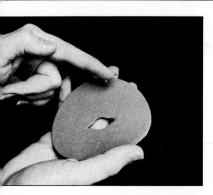

2 Next, moisten the Colly-Seel ring with warm tap water. Rub water into the ring until it becomes sticky.
Knead the moistened ring to make it more flexible. Or, warm it between your hands. A flexible ring fits better around the drain.

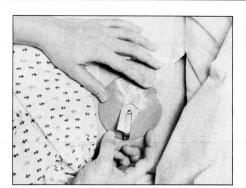

3 Now, center the ring over your patient's drain, as the nurse is doing here. Gently press the ring onto the skin, smoothing out any wrinkles or bubbles.

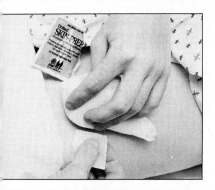

2 Are you using individual disposable wipes saturated in Skin-Prep? If so, open the package and use the wipe to swab the area around the drain. Make sure you've covered the skin completely. Then, let it dry for approximately 30 seconds.

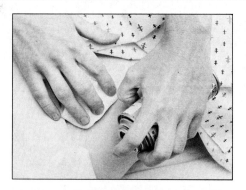

3 To use Skin-Prep aerosol, spray around the wound and drain evenly. Let it dry for about 30 seconds. *Important:* Never spray Skin-Prep directly onto a wound.

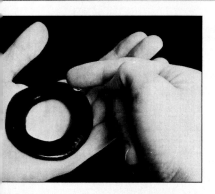

2 Slightly moisten the karaya seal with a few drops of warm water until it becomes sticky. Now, you can easily shape the ring to fit the drain's dimensions.

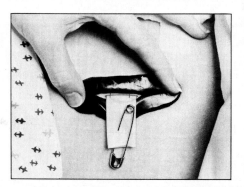

3 Then, place the seal around your patient's drain, making sure it fits snugly at the base. Gently press the seal so it adheres to the skin.
Suppose you're using karaya powder. Sprinkle it on the skin surrounding the drain. To prevent irritation or infection, avoid getting the powder in the wound.

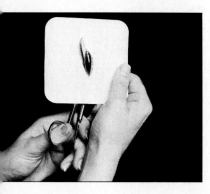

2 Cut an opening the same size as the drain and remove the Stomahesive backing.

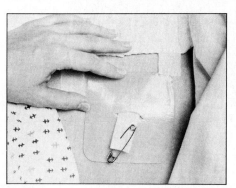

3 Center the sheet, sticky side down, over your patient's drain. Gently press the sheet on his skin, smoothing out any wrinkles. Hold the Stomahesive in place for 30 seconds, until it's stabilized.

Draining wounds

Applying skin barriers continued

Applying ReliaSeal™

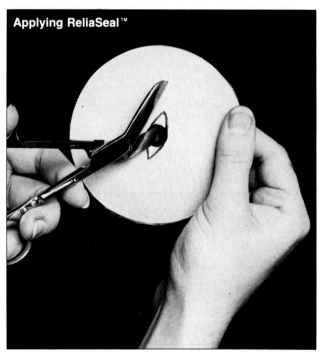

1 If you're applying ReliaSeal skin barrier, cut an opening the same size as your patient's drain.

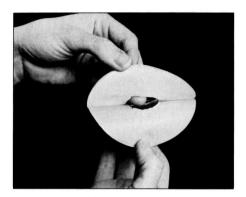

2 Next, remove the white paper covering the Relia-Seal, as shown here.

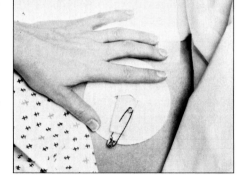

3 Center the ReliaSeal over your patient's drain, and press gently to remove all wrinkles.

After a few minutes, your patient's body heat will soften the protective gel against his skin. This will secure the seal.

If you're applying a drainage pouch over the ReliaSeal, peel off the ReliaSeal's blue paper backing. The adhesive underneath this backing will secure the pouch to the seal.

Applying zinc oxide

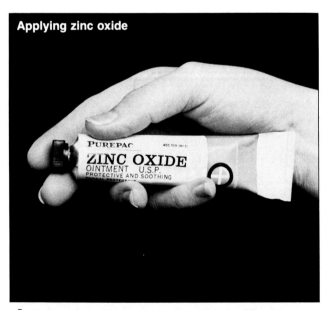

1 Unlike other skin barriers, zinc oxide is difficult to remove from the patient's skin. Avoid using this ointment when the skin surrounding your patient's wound is tender and sore. And *never* apply it to the wound itself.

To apply zinc oxide, wash your hands and put on a pair of gloves.

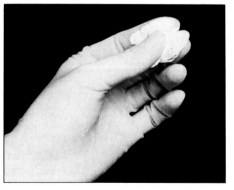

2 Remove a generous amount of the ointment from the container. Warm the cream by rubbing it between your gloved fingers.

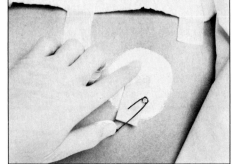

3 Begin applying the skin barrier at the drain and work outward. Using a clean gauze pad, apply downward strokes to remove excess cream.

Remove your gloves.

Applying a disposable pouch

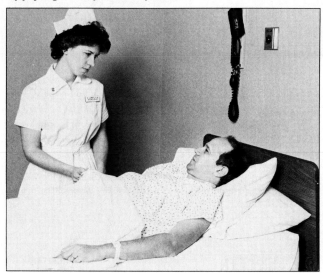

1 *Picture this: Avery Cook, a 38-year-old cab driver, has just returned to your unit from surgery to remove the head of his pancreas. Because the doctor anticipates a large amount of wound drainage, he made a small incision and inserted a Penrose drain parallel to the suture line. Now, to prevent the need for frequent dressing changes, the doctor asks you to apply a disposable pouch over the drain. Do you know how? If you're unsure, follow these guidelines:*

Begin by gathering the equipment you'll need: a drainable disposable pouch with adhesive square; a skin barrier (such as Colly-Seel), if you feel the patient needs the extra protection this affords; pouch closure or rubber band; measuring card or pattern; nonallergenic tape; scissors; and a plastic bag.

Explain the procedure to Mr. Cook, even if he seems groggy. Expose the area around his wound. Drape his body to keep him warm and ensure his privacy.

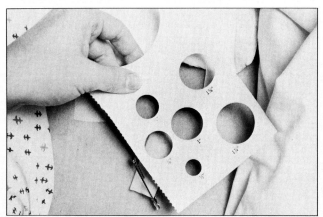

2 Wash your hands and remove the soiled dressing. Discard it in the plastic bag. Wash your hands again. Now, using the measuring card or pattern, determine the size of Mr. Cook's drain by centering one of the larger circles over it. If the circle's too large, try smaller circles until you find the one that's the right size.

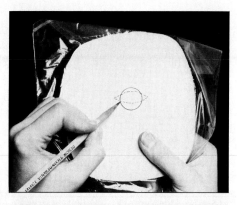

3 Next, trace the pattern onto the pouch's adhesive square.

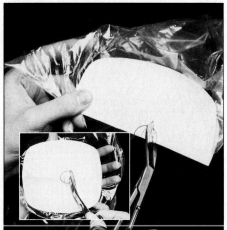

4 Fold the adhesive backing in half, lengthwise. Cut the pattern in the adhesive, as the nurse is doing here. To prevent cutting through the pouch, keep the pouch away from the adhesive. (If the pouch has a precut opening, make sure the opening is the proper size.)

📨 *Nursing tip:* If the pouch you plan to use has a large opening in the bottom, you can keep the pouch away from the adhesive by slipping your hand up through the pouch and spreading your fingers behind the adhesive (see inset).

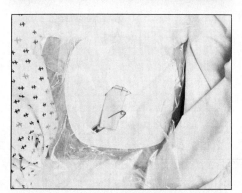

5 Now, peel off the backing from the adhesive seal. Center the pouch's opening over your patient's drain. Gently press down the seal, taking care to smooth out any wrinkles with your fingers.

📨 *Nursing tip:* Place a 4"x4" gauze pad over the drain to absorb excess fluids while you apply the bag. Remove it before the bag is completely applied.

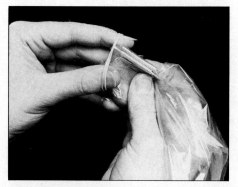

6 To close your patient's pouch, turn up the bottom two or three times; then fanfold the end of it sideways.

Tightly wrap a rubber band around the end of the pouch, as shown here. Or, attach a clamp, such as the Hollister drainable pouch clamp, to the bottom.

Finally, document the entire procedure in your nurses' notes.

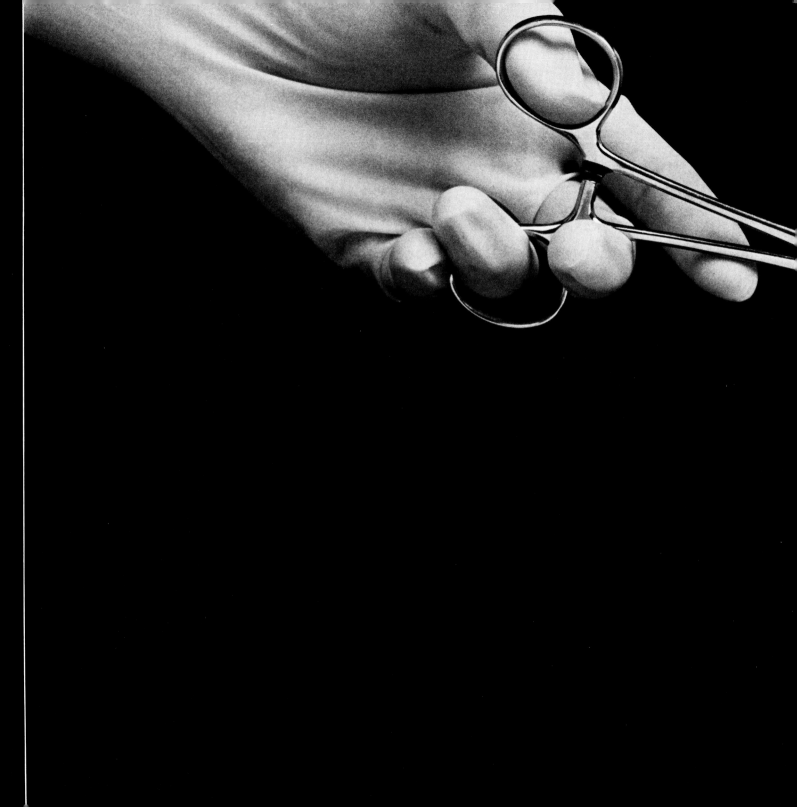

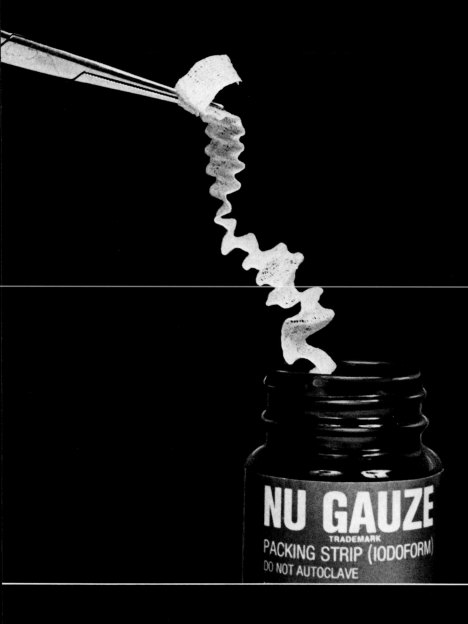

Dealing with Complications

Respiratory problems

Wound management

Special considerations

NU GAUZE
TRADEMARK
PACKING STRIP (IODOFORM)
DO NOT AUTOCLAVE

Respiratory problems

Before your patient underwent surgery, you worked hard to protect him from possible postop respiratory complications. You taught him deep breathing and coughing exercises, and acquainted him with incentive spirometry. Then, after surgery, you conscientiously helped him perform his exercises on a regular basis.

But, despite your best efforts, your patient may still develop a respiratory complication—especially if he's a high-risk patient. If he does, can you recognize early signs and symptoms? Do you know what action to take? Read the following pages to find out.

Note: For more information, review pages 34 to 43 of this book. In addition, consult the NURSING PHOTOBOOK PROVIDING RESPIRATORY CARE.

Nurses' guide to respiratory complications

If your patient's had major surgery, he faces the risk of developing one of the respiratory complications described here. Safeguard your patient by making sure you can quickly recognize a developing problem; then, take appropriate action.

If your patient develops any respiratory complication, monitor his condition by frequently auscultating his breath sounds. In addition, regularly assess his arterial blood gas measurements for early signs of hypoxia. If hypoxia develops, be prepared to administer oxygen, as ordered. (For more information on hypoxia, refer to page 144.)

Equally important, provide extra emotional support for your patient. Remember, he's likely to be frightened by his breathing difficulties. Take special care to explain all procedures to him, and to answer his questions.

Finally, document all procedures, as well as your observations, in your nurses' notes.

Now, read this chart for details on specific respiratory complications.

Complication	Contributing factors
Atelectasis (Incomplete expansion of alveoli or lung segments, which may result in partial or total lung collapse. After surgery, this is usually caused by excessive secretions or a mucus plug.)	• Administration of gas anesthetics with high oxygen and low nitrogen concentrations • Prolonged intubation of left or right mainstem bronchus, which predisposes lung on opposite side to atelectasis • Inadequate suctioning during intubation, allowing bronchial secretions to accumulate • Suppression of cough reflex by sedatives or anesthetics • Failure to adequately deep breathe and cough following abdominal or thoracic surgery, from incisional pain or a tight-fitting dressing • Dehydration • Prolonged immobilization after surgery • Impaired alveolar function; from chronic obstructive pulmonary disease (COPD), for example • Weak respiratory muscles • Elevated diaphragm; from abdominal gas, bleeding, or tumor, for example
Pneumonia (Lung inflammation with consolidation)	• Aspiration of foreign material; for example, vomitus • Infection • Atelectasis • Chemical inhalation • Prolonged immobilization after surgery • Dehydration • Failure to adequately deep breathe and cough after abdominal or thoracic surgery • Suppression of cough reflex by sedatives or anesthetics • Impaired alveolar function • Weak respiratory muscles
Pulmonary embolism (Obstruction of pulmonary arterial bed by dislodged thrombus)	• Prolonged immobility • Thrombophlebitis • Chronic pulmonary disease • Chronic atrial fibrillation • Lower extremity fracture • Use of oral contraceptives • Advanced age • Sickle cell anemia

Signs and symptoms	Nursing interventions
• Dyspnea and cyanosis • Tachycardia • Diminished or absent breath sounds on auscultation • Flatness on percussion • Decreased chest expansion • Decreased blood pressure • Increased temperature • Restlessness • Confusion	• Encourage patient to deep breathe frequently, using the principles of sustained maximal inspiration described on page 34, and to cough. • Administer prophylactic antibiotics, if ordered. • Administer humidified air or oxygen, with or without a mucolytic drug, to loosen secretions, as ordered. • If ordered, use chest percussion (or vibration) along with postural drainage to help clear secretions. To encourage gravitational drainage, position the patient so the affected lung area is elevated above unaffected areas. (See page 128 for details on chest physiotherapy.) • Using clean technique, perform nasotracheal suctioning, if needed. (This procedure may require a doctor's order, so check your hospital's policy.) • Prepare the patient for possible deep suctioning by bronchoscopy, a procedure performed by the doctor. • Administer intermittent positive pressure breathing (IPPB) therapy, if ordered (see pages 42 to 43). • Begin mechanical ventilation, if ordered.
• Sudden onset of shaking chills • Fever • Flushed skin • Cough with production of pinkish or rust-colored sputum • Sharp chest pain in lateral lung fields; increased pain on inspiration • Headache • Rales or rhonchi • Tachypnea • Decreased breath sounds from affected lung area	• Periodically obtain sputum for culture and sensitivity. To prevent spread of infection, dispose of secretions according to your hospital's infection control standards. • Encourage the patient to avoid dehydration by drinking plenty of fluids. • Encourage the patient to frequently deep breathe and cough. • Administer antibiotics, if ordered. • If ordered, use chest percussion (or vibration) along with postural drainage to help clear secretions. • Administer humidified air or oxygen, with or without a mucolytic drug, to loosen secretions (as ordered). • Using clean technique, perform nasotracheal suctioning, if needed. (This procedure may require a doctor's order.) • Conserve the patient's energy by providing adequate rest; remember, he may become easily exhausted.
• Dyspnea • Tachycardia • Anginal or pleuritic chest pain • Pleuritic (pleural) friction rub • Productive cough (sputum may be blood-tinged) • Low-grade fever • Cyanosis • Syncope • Neck vein distention • Restlessness • Massive hemoptysis (rarely)	• Administer oxygen by face mask or nasal cannula, as ordered. • Be prepared to intubate the patient, if necessary. • Prepare the patient for a chest X-ray and lung scan. • Connect patient to a cardiac monitor, or obtain frequent EKGs. • Implement anticoagulant drug therapy, as ordered. *Important:* Before administering an anticoagulant drug, find out which other drugs your patient's taking, and how they interact with the prescribed anticoagulant. If the doctor's ordered heparin sodium (Lipo-Hepin), have protamine sulfate on hand to neutralize the heparin sodium, if necessary. • Obtain blood coagulation studies and closely monitor them. • Elevate head of bed to relieve dyspnea. • Monitor arterial blood gas measurements, as ordered. • Monitor fluid intake and output. Insert an indwelling (Foley) catheter, if ordered. • Administer an analgesic, as ordered, to relieve pain and anxiety. • Conserve the patient's energy by providing adequate rest.

Respiratory problems

Understanding chest physiotherapy

You can use chest physiotherapy techniques to prevent or treat your postoperative patient's respiratory problems. For example, the doctor may order it if your patient's on prolonged bed rest, or if he's developed atelectasis or pneumonia. (For details on recognizing respiratory complications, read the chart on the preceding pages.)

The three techniques described here are most effective when performed together. Explain the procedure to the patient and his family before you begin.

POSTURAL DRAINAGE

Purpose
Postural drainage enables pulmonary secretions to drain by gravity into the major bronchi or the trachea. Then, your patient can dislodge them by coughing. If he can't, he may need percussion and/or vibration techniques.

Procedure
• Place the lung segment to be drained uppermost, with the mainstem bronchus as close to vertical as possible. Remember, positions for postural drainage vary, depending on which lung segment's involved.

Nursing considerations
• Don't perform postural drainage immediately after the patient eats.
• When you drain lower lobes, decrease the drainage angle if your patient can't tolerate the necessary angle (for example, if he has chronic obstructive pulmonary disease).
• Don't use Trendelenberg position if your patient has increased intracranial pressure or acute heart disease, or has had major abdominal or brain surgery.
• Monitor your patient's cardiac and respiratory status during treatment.
Note: For more information on postural drainage, see the NURSING PHOTOBOOK PROVIDING RESPIRATORY CARE.

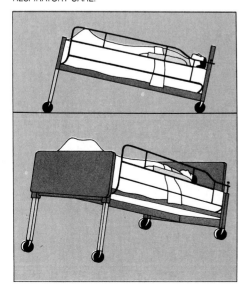

PERCUSSION

Purpose
Percussion mechanically dislodges thick, tenacious secretions from the bronchial walls so they can be expectorated or suctioned.

Procedure
• Hold your hands in a cupped shape. Keep your fingers flexed and your thumb tight against your index finger.
• Percuss the chest segment you're draining by alternating your hands in a rhythmic manner. For the technique to work effectively, you must trap air between your hand and the patient's chest. You should hear a hollow sound when doing the procedure—not a loud slap.

Nursing considerations
• Always have a towel, sheet, or patient gown between your hands and the patient's skin. Percuss for 3 to 5 minutes while your patient's in each postural drainage position.
• Don't percuss over your patient's spine or sternum, or below his thoracic cage.
• Avoid percussion if your patient has rib or spinal fractures, flail chest or other traumatic chest injury, pulmonary hemorrhage, pulmonary embolus, mastectomy with silicone implant, metastatic lesion of ribs, pneumothorax, or hemothorax.

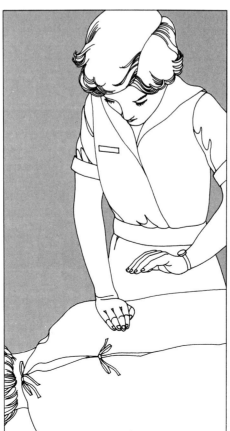

VIBRATION

Purpose
Vibration increases velocity and turbulence of exhaled air. This loosens secretions and helps propel them into the larger bronchi so they can be expectorated or suctioned.

Procedure
• Place your hands flat (side by side with your fingers extended) on the chest segment you're draining.
• Instruct your patient to inhale deeply. Then, as he *slowly* exhales, vibrate his chest by quickly contracting and relaxing the muscles of your arms and shoulders. Stop vibrating when he inhales again. Repeat this procedure several times.

Nursing considerations
• Use vibration instead of percussion if your patient has extreme pain in chest area, is frail, or has just had thoracic surgery.
• Vibrate your patient's chest in each postural drainage position. If the doctor orders, alternate this method with percussion.
• Don't vibrate over your patient's spine or sternum, or below his thoracic cage.
• Avoid pressing hard on the patient's ribs, since this may be painful.
• Try to synchronize vibrations with patient's exhalations.
  Nursing tip: Consider using a specially-designed electric vibrator (if available) to produce the same effect.

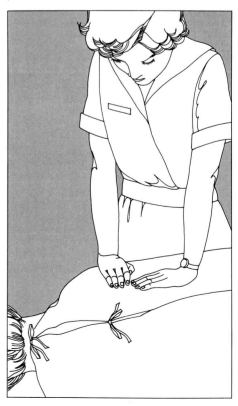

Wound management

How skilled are you at caring for a patient with a wound complication? For example, do you know how to recognize the signs and symptoms? How to identify possible causes? How to manage the problem? How to prevent further complications?

On the pages that follow, we'll answer these questions. In addition, you'll find step-by-step guidelines for:
• obtaining aerobic and anaerobic wound cultures.
• applying a warm, wet compress.
• irrigating and packing your patient's wound.
• applying a scultetus or a Velcro abdominal binder.

Recognizing wound complications

Are you caring for a patient who's recently returned from surgery? As you know, part of postop assessment involves inspecting your patient's dressing and wound. Do this every 30 minutes for the first 2 hours. After the initial postoperative period, check your patient's dressing and wound every 2 hours, or as indicated.

As you assess your patient's dressing and wound, note the color and amount of blood or drainage (if any). Remember, some blood and drainage is considered normal. However, if the bleeding becomes profuse or the drainage purulent, notify the doctor. Also, be sure that the sutures (if any) are in place and that the wound is pink, with no signs of inflammation. Document your findings, including the time and date, in your nurses' notes.

Keep in mind, though, that wound complications may develop suddenly, causing a serious setback in your patient's condition. Learn how to recognize some of the more common wound complications, and how to cope with them.

Study the chart below carefully. Remember—your ability to make accurate, quick observations may prevent a full-fledged crisis.

HEMORRHAGE

Possible causes
• Slipped suture
• Dislodged blood clot
• Sloughing of blood clot
• Infection
• Accidental surgical nick of blood vessel
• Blood vessel erosion, possibly caused by a drain or packing
• Underlying blood-clotting disorder

Signs and symptoms
• Steady blood flow from wound
• Hypovolemic shock (rapid pulse, shallow respirations, pallor, cold perspiration, restlessness, and irritability)

Nursing considerations
• Place the patient in Trendelenberg position, unless contraindicated.
• Stay with your patient while someone else notifies the doctor.
• If bleeding is profuse, apply pressure to wound until doctor arrives.
• Prepare to assist the doctor in suture application. (The patient's wound may require surgical repair in the operating room.)
• Check number of blood units on hold. Consider emergency type and crossmatch.
• Prevent further complications; for example, aspiration of blood after face or dental surgery.
• Prepare equipment to start an I.V., if one isn't already in place.

DEHISCENCE AND EVISCERATION

Possible causes
• Infection at wound site, causing tissue degeneration and slippage of sutures
• Failure of deep wound tissues to unite
• Poor wound healing, caused, for example, by malnutrition
• Abdominal distention from paralytic ileus or intestinal obstruction

Signs and symptoms
• Low-grade fever, with no apparent cause, lasting 3 to 4 days
• Prolonged, increasing, or severe pain at wound site 3 to 4 days after surgery
• Pinkish-clear fluid saturating dressing
• Partial or total separation of wound edges (dehiscence)
• Patient may experience feeling of giving way or pulling apart at suture line.

• Sudden, dramatic bursting of suture line, with abdominal contents protruding from gap (evisceration)

Nursing considerations
• Notify doctor immediately. These complications may be life-threatening. *Important:* Don't leave your patient alone. If necessary, ask a co-worker to notify the doctor while you care for your patient.
• If dehiscence occurs, consider applying a binder to provide support for the wound.
• If evisceration occurs, do not reinsert abdominal contents. Instead, cover them with gauze pads or sterile towels saturated with normal saline solution.
• Keep patient in supine position.
• If possible, move patient to quiet area to keep him from becoming more anxious.
• Discourage coughing or any maneuver that may increase intra-abdominal pressure.
• Prepare patient for surgery to close wound, as ordered.

HEMATOMA

Possible cause
• Bleeding and clot formation in wound

Signs and symptoms
• Ecchymotic area on skin surface or at suture site
• Bulging from wound or suture site, suggesting deep hematoma
• Pain at wound site

Nursing considerations
• If you observe a small hematoma at the wound site, closely monitor its size. If it increases in size, notify the doctor.
• Be prepared to assist doctor with hematoma removal, if necessary.
• After hematoma removal, frequently check the patient for bleeding. If bleeding is present, notify the doctor. He may cauterize small bleeding vessels, or place additional sutures in the wound.

Wound management

Recognizing wound complications continued

INCISIONAL INFECTION

Possible cause
• Poor aseptic technique before, during, or after surgery, allowing infecting organisms such as *Staphylococcus aureus* and microaerophilic streptococci to enter the incision

Signs and symptoms
• Elevated or decreased temperature
• Elevated pulse rate
• Induration around incision
• Warmth, tenderness, redness, and swelling at incision site
• Purulent drainage from incision (varying in color, odor, and consistency)
• Severe pain at incision site
• Headache
• Nausea, vomiting
• Generalized swelling and tenderness of lymph nodes
• Weakness, malaise

Nursing considerations
• Place patient in either wound and skin isolation or strict isolation, to prevent spread of infection. *Important:* If your patient's not isolated, you may isolate his soiled dressing or implement modified wound isolation without a doctor's order.
• Obtain aerobic and anaerobic cultures, as ordered.
• Obtain an order to apply warm compresses to the wound site; warm compresses relieve pain, diminish spasms and increase blood flow and lymphatic drainage.
• Be ready to administer a broad-spectrum antibiotic such as cephalothin sodium (Keflin Neutral*), I.V., as ordered.
• Elevate infected area, if possible, to reduce swelling and improve venous and lymphatic drainage.
• Observe for signs and symptoms of gas gangrene (ecchymosis, crepitus, and foul odor), especially in a patient who's undergone extensive bowel surgery, or one who's suffered traumatic injury.
• Observe incision for signs of a healing ridge (palpable in 4 to 5 days). If a ridge doesn't develop, dehiscence may occur. Notify the doctor.
• Monitor fluid intake and output. Remember, if the patient has a fever, he'll need more fluids.
• Maintain nutritional support to help fight infection and promote tissue healing. Total parenteral nutrition (TPN) may be necessary.

DEEP WOUND INFECTION

Possible cause
• Preexisting infection; for example, peritonitis from ruptured appendix or diverticulum
• Accidental surgical nick of stomach, intestinal tract, or gall bladder

Signs and symptoms
• Elevated temperature
• Elevated pulse
• Warmth, swelling, tenderness, and redness over the infection site
• Induration around infection site
• Possible purulent drainage, if a drain is located at infection site
• Severe pain at infection site, especially if a large abcess is pressing on nerve endings
• Anorexia, nausea, vomiting
• Profound malaise and weakness
  Important: Signs and symptoms of wound infection may be masked by the action of previously-administered antibiotics.

Nursing considerations
• Isolate the patient if the infection site is draining.
• *Don't* apply warm compresses or any other heat source to the area. This may cause a well-encapsulated abcess in the abdominal or thoracic cavity to burst.
• Obtain aerobic and anaerobic wound cultures, as ordered, if the infection site is draining.
• Be prepared to assist the doctor with needle aspiration of suppurant, if the infection site has no external opening.
• If necessary, remind the doctor of any antibiotics the patient is presently receiving. The doctor may temporarily stop antibiotic administration and order reculturing, to identify causative organisms.
• Obtain blood cultures, if ordered.
• Observe for signs of gas gangrene, especially in a patient who's undergone extensive bowel surgery, or one who's suffered traumatic injury.
• Prepare your patient for extensive X-ray tests (for example, gallium scans), to determine the location and size of the infection.
• Monitor the patient's fluid intake and output, and maintain adequate intake. Fever increases your patient's fluid needs. In addition, some abcesses sequester fluids inside themselves, which also increases fluid needs.
• Consider using TPN to help meet your patient's metabolic needs.

*Available in both the United States and in Canada

Obtaining an aerobic wound culture

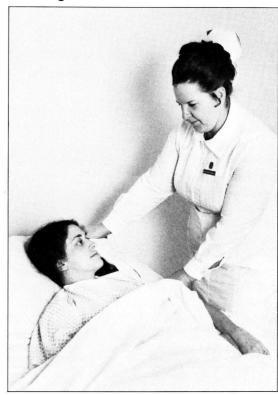

1 *Thirty-four-year-old Bernadette Chinskey is recovering from surgery. Today, her abdominal surgical wound dehisced, as the result of a deep wound infection. The doctor expects you to take an aerobic culture to determine the infection's cause. Here's how to proceed:*

Begin by assembling this sterile equipment: culture swab with culture medium (such as Culturette® II), two packages of 4"x4" gauze pads, gloves, normal saline solution or water, and basin.

Then, explain the procedure to Ms. Chinskey. Remove the dressing to expose her wound. Wash your hands thoroughly.

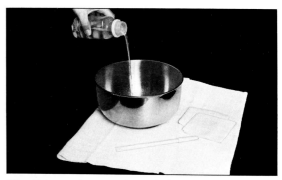

2 Using strict aseptic technique, open your sterile supplies. Pour saline solution into the basin, as shown here.

Next, put on your gloves.

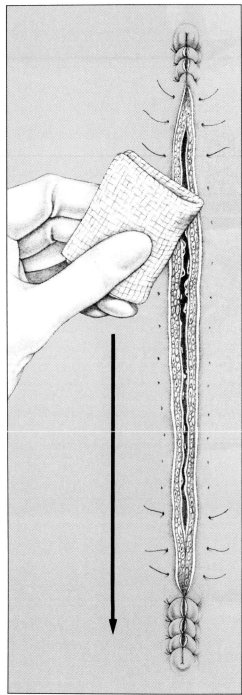

3 Carefully clean the wound with a gauze pad moistened in the saline solution. Wipe from top to bottom and discard the pad. Using another pad saturated with solution, repeat this procedure until you've removed all the gross external debris. By doing so, you remove superficial microorganisms that may contaminate the culture. Dry the wound with a dry gauze pad.

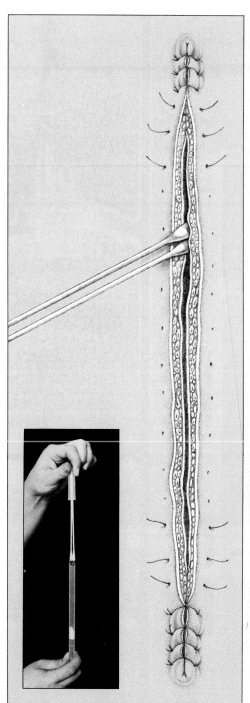

4 Remove your gloves. Holding the Culturette at its base, remove the applicator swab (see inset photo). Position the swab in the wound at the site of the most drainage. Collect as much drainage as possible. *Important:* Be sure the specimen you collect comes from inside the wound. A surface specimen may alter the accuracy of the lab analysis.

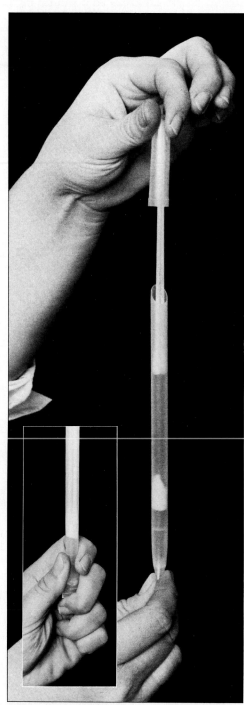

5 Return the swab to its container, as shown. Now, crush the culture-medium ampule at the base of the tube and push the swab into the medium (see inset photo). Wash your hands. Label the specimen and appropriate lab slip. Remember to request a sensitivity test, if ordered. Send the specimen to the lab immediately. Document what you've done.

Wound management

How to obtain an anaerobic wound culture

1 *Do you know how to collect an anaerobic specimen? Keep in mind that you can collect anaerobic and aerobic specimens at the same time or separately. If you're using an Anaerobic Culturette®, like the one illustrated at right, follow these steps:*

Gather the necessary sterile equipment: 4"x4" gauze pads, normal saline solution, basin, and gloves. You'll also need an Anaerobic Culturette.

Now, tell your patient what you're going to do. Wash your hands. Remove the dressing, and wash your hands again.

Using aseptic technique, open all your supplies and put on your gloves. Clean the wound, using the same procedure shown on page 131. Remove the sterile gloves. *Note:* If you need to separate the wound edges to obtain the specimen, leave on your gloves. However, take care not to contaminate any part of the Culturette with your gloves after you've touched the wound. Doing so could spread infection.

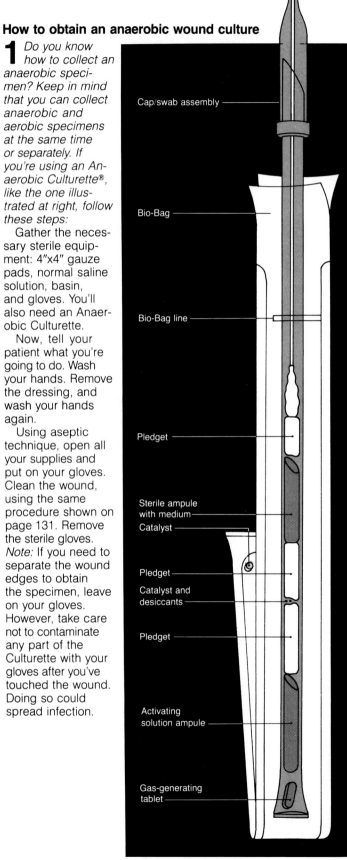

Cap/swab assembly

Bio-Bag

Bio-Bag line

Pledget

Sterile ampule with medium

Catalyst

Pledget

Catalyst and desiccants

Pledget

Activating solution ampule

Gas-generating tablet

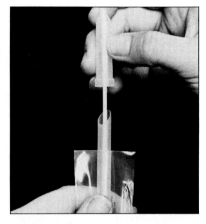

2 Peel open the Culturette package and remove the Culturette and Bio-Bag. Then, remove the Culturette cap and attached swab, as shown.

Next, insert the swab into the wound at the site that has the most drainage. Insert the swab as deeply as you can without hurting the patient. Collect as much drainage as possible.

Put the cap back on the Culturette tube, and gently push the tube into the Bio-Bag until the top of the cap reaches the bag's line.

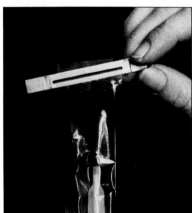

3 To fasten the bag, remove the metal closure from under the bag's label. Slip the top of the Bio-Bag through the metal closure, as shown here. Then, fold the top of the bag over the closure at least three times, until the closure reaches the line. Bend the closure ends so they are opposite the direction of the fold.

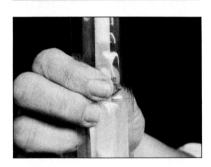

4 Invert the Bio-Bag so the Culturette cap is facing down. Crush the ampule next to the swab with your fingers, as shown here.

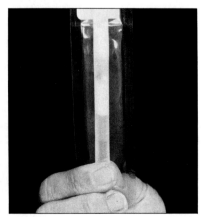

5 Now, invert the Bio-Bag so the Culturette cap is facing upward. Using your fingers, crush the bottom ampule. Continue holding the Bio-Bag upright until the tablet's completely dissolved and the Bio-Bag inflates.

Wash your hands. Label the Bio-Bag and lab slip. Request a sensitivity test, if ordered. Send the Bio-Bag to the lab, and document the procedure.

Using a Curity® heating unit

1 *Consider this situation: The doctor has ordered the application of warm, wet compresses over your patient's infected surgical wound to encourage purulent secretions to drain. You'll apply a compress once every 2 to 4 hours, leaving each compress in place for approximately 20 minutes. If you have a Curity heating unit, follow these steps:*

First, gather the equipment you need: several packages of Curity wet dressings premoistened with sterile saline solution or distilled water (depending on the doctor's order), 5"x9" dry dressing, sterile gloves, the heating unit, and nonallergenic tape (not shown). If you must remove a soiled dressing before applying the wet compress, also obtain nonsterile gloves and a plastic bag. Place the equipment on a bedside table. *Important:* Keep the heater away from flammable items, such as bed linen or curtains. And, if your patient's receiving oxygen, turn it off before using the heater. Or, if your patient can't comfortably tolerate this, operate the heater in a safer place, such as a clean utility room.

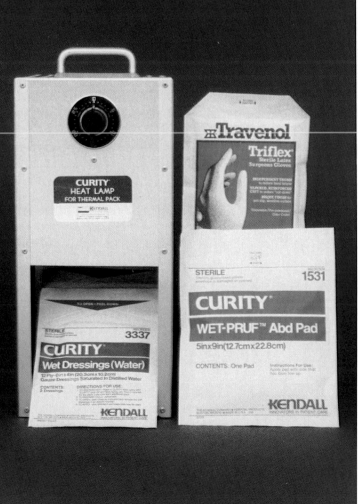

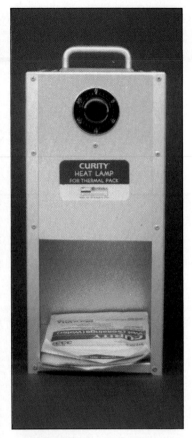

2 Next, plug in the heater and set the power switch to the ON position. To determine the proper heating time, allow 5 minutes to heat the top pad, and 3 minutes to heat each additional pad. Set the timer dial for the appropriate time period. Since this nurse is heating two pads, she set the timer for 8 minutes.

Without unwrapping the compresses, place them in the heater, as shown here, with the peel flaps facing out. If the compresses are moistened with distilled water, like the ones shown here, place the pads so their labels face up. If they're moistened with saline solution, place the pads so their labels face down. (You may place up to six pads in the heater. The number depends on the wound's size.)

While the compresses are heating, put on nonsterile gloves and remove your patient's soiled dressings. Then, remove your soiled gloves and properly dispose of all soiled equipment. Wash and dry your hands.

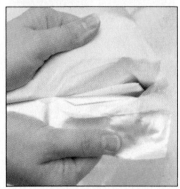

3 When the time you've set has expired, the heater will automatically turn off. After this happens, take a compress package from the heater and open it, peeling the foil wrapping back with both hands. Make sure you don't touch the sterile pad. Leaving the pad on its sterile wrapper, lay it on a clean, dry surface. Open the other pad in the same way. Then, put on your sterile gloves.

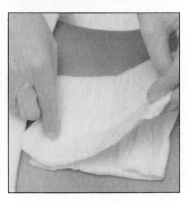

4 Lift the compress from its wrapping and place it over your patient's wound, as shown here. Repeat the procedure to apply the second compress.

Wound management

Using a Curity® heating unit continued

5 Cover the wet dressing with the 5"x9" dry dressing. Secure it with nonallergenic tape or Montgomery straps. Document the procedure and your observations.

Remove the compresses after about 20 minutes, since they cool quickly. Properly dispose of the soiled compresses, and re-dress the wound with another sterile dry dressing.

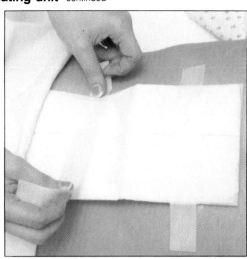

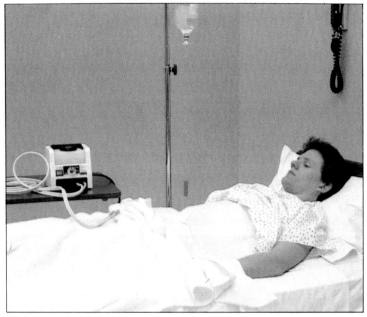

6 If the doctor orders continuous warm, wet compresses for your patient, you'll need a disposable water circulation heating pad and heating module (such as the American™ Duo-Therm™ disposable pad or K®-pad, and Aquamatic K®-module), and a sterile barrier.

First, fill the heating module's water reservoir with distilled water. Then, attach the reservoir tubing to the disposable heating pad. Make sure the connection is secure.

Plug the module into an electrical outlet. Use the key provided with the module to set the correct temperature, as ordered by the doctor. Allow at least 1½ minutes for the pad to heat.

To prevent the heating pad from contaminating the sterile dressing, place a sterile barrier over the patient's dressing. Then, lay the heating pad over the sterile barrier, as shown here. Continue the treatment for the ordered length of time. Frequently check the patient's skin for signs of burns.

Document the entire procedure, as well as your observations, in your nurses' notes.

How to make a warm, wet compress

1 *If you don't have a Curity heating unit, make your own warm, wet compresses. Read this photostory to learn how.*

You'll need this sterile equipment: normal saline solution or distilled water (depending on the doctor's order), a small basin, 4"x4" gauze pads, gloves, and a Surgipad (not shown). You'll also need a clean bath basin, several towels, and nonallergenic tape (not shown).

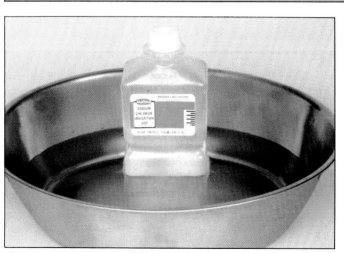

2 Half-fill the bath basin with hot tap water. Place the bottle of normal saline solution into the hot water for about 30 minutes. (Replace the water as often as necessary to keep it hot.)

☎ *Nursing tip:* If you prefer, place the solution bottle in a small metal bath basin half-filled with water, and heat the water on an electric hot plate, until it's 105° F. (41° C.).

When the solution's been warming for 30 minutes, remove your patient's soiled dressing.

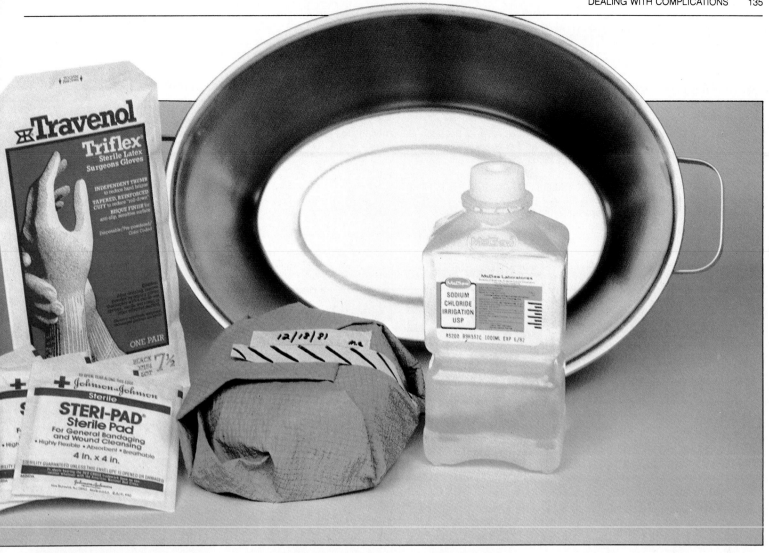

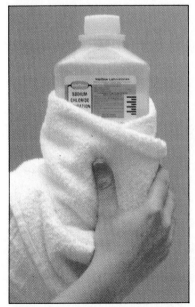

3 Next, remove the bottle from the basin. Wrap a towel around the bottle, so you can handle it comfortably.

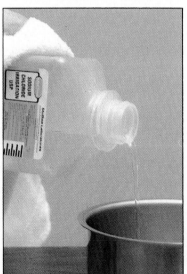

4 Open the solution bottle and pour some of the solution into the sterile bowl, as shown. Then, open the packs of sterile gauze pads, using strict aseptic technique.

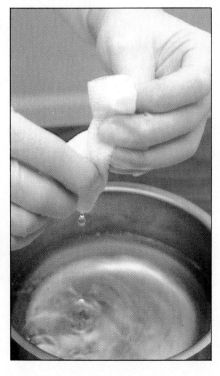

5 Now, put on sterile gloves. Pick up one of the gauze pads and dip it into the solution. Twist the pad over the basin to squeeze out any excess solution, as shown.

Place the pad over the patient's wound. Repeat this procedure until the wound's completely covered.

Place a Surgipad over the wet dressing and secure the dressing with nonallergenic tape or Montgomery straps. *Remember:* Leave the dressing in place for only about 20 minutes, or as ordered.

Document the procedure in your nurses' notes.

Wound management

Applying a scultetus binder

1 *Consider this situation: Mildred Sero, a 30-year-old newspaper reporter, is recovering from exploratory abdominal surgery. While you're changing her dressing, you notice several eroded sutures. To provide wide abdominal support and prevent wound dehiscence, you prepare to apply a scultetus binder. Here's how to proceed:*

First, explain the procedure to the patient. Tell her that the binder will support her incision, and make her more comfortable.

Now, turn her to one side. (Remember to help her splint her incision as she turns.) Fanfold the binder under her. Then, turn her to her opposite side and unfold the binder.

Next, position her on her back in the center of the binder, as shown here, with her body well-aligned. Check to be sure that the top of the binder is at about waist level.

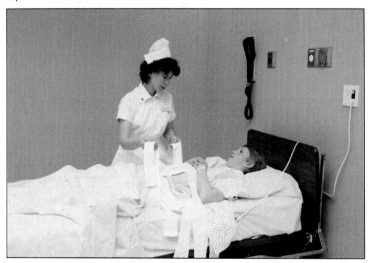

2 Now, you're ready to begin closing the binder. To do so, use your left hand to bring the bottom tail at Ms. Sero's left side to the center of her abdomen. Maintaining tension on the left tail, overlap it with the right tail. Repeat the procedure on the next pair of tails, as shown. *Note:* If your patient is small or thin, like Ms. Sero, double the tails back on themselves, as the nurse is doing here. However, don't allow the thicker seamed edges to press on any pressure points, such as her hips.

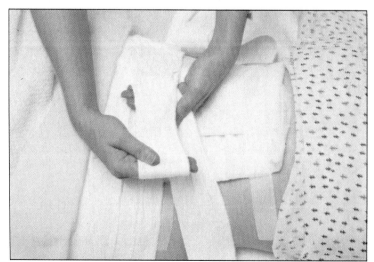

3 Working upward, continue bringing each left tail to the center, and overlap it with the opposite tail on the right. As you work, make sure each pair of tails overlaps the pair below, as shown here.

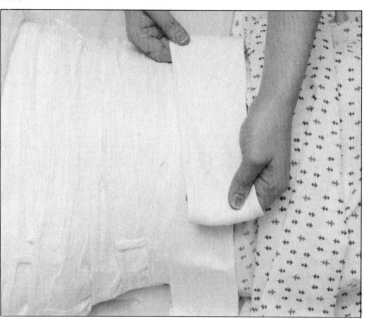

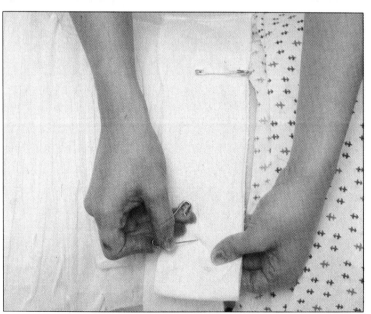

4 Finally, secure the top pair of tails with safety pins, as the nurse is doing here. Or, secure the tails with tape.

Check to be sure Ms. Sero can breathe easily and that the binder feels comfortable. The binder should be snug enough to effectively support the incision, but not so tight that it inhibits deep breathing and coughing. If necessary, loosen the binder appropriately.

Document the procedure in your nurses' notes. Remove the binder as necessary to assess the wound. When you do so, check the patient's skin for signs of irritation or developing pressure sores.

Applying a Velcro® binder

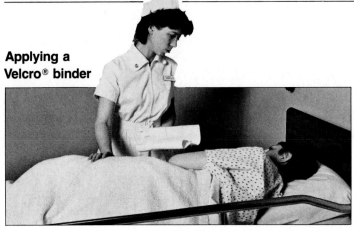

1 *Suppose you're supporting Ms. Sero's incision with a Velcro binder; for example, the Flexitone® DUO™ Surgical binder featured here. Follow these steps:*

Help Ms. Sero to turn onto her side. (Splint her incision as she turns, if she's unable to do so herself.) Remember to explain why you're applying a binder. Then, fanfold the binder and place it behind her.

2 Turn your patient to her other side and position the binder under her, as in the previous photostory. Then, place her on her back in the center of the binder. Check to be sure that the top of the binder is at about waist level, as shown.

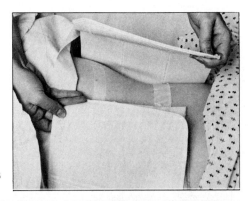

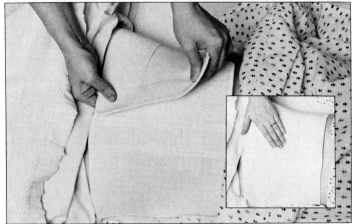

3 To close the binder, pull the left end toward the center of Ms. Sero's abdomen. As you maintain tension on the left end, pull the right end over the left, as the nurse is doing here.

[Inset] Then, secure both ends by smoothing the Velcro edges together. Ask Ms. Sero if the binder feels comfortable. If she complains of tightness or breathing difficulties, loosen the binder accordingly.

Document the procedure and the type of binder used in your nurses' notes. As necessary, remove the binder to observe the patient's wound. When you do so, check her skin for signs of irritation or developing pressure sores.

Irrigating and packing a wound

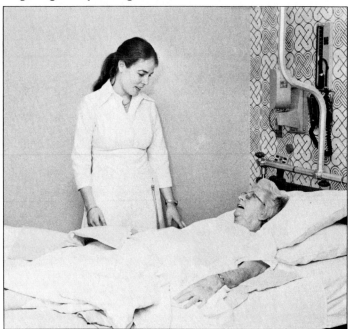

1 *Evelyn Woodard, a 62-year-old housewife, has undergone a vulvectomy to remove a cancerous tumor. The doctor expects you to irrigate her open surgical wound, apply fibrinolysin and desoxyribonuclease ointment (Elase*), and pack the wound with gauze soaked in povidone-iodine solution. This procedure helps debride the wound, and promotes healing from the inside. Do you know how to proceed? Read on.*

First, gather the necessary clean equipment: irrigating solution composed of half hydrogen peroxide and half normal saline solution (as ordered), povidone-iodine solution, normal saline solution, several 4"x4" gauze pads, basin, scissors, forceps, Surgipad, bed-saver pads or an emesis basin, Elase ointment, and a roll of Kling™ gauze.

You'll also need two pairs of nonsterile gloves, nonallergenic tape, and a plastic bag to dispose of soiled dressings and equipment. Observe clean technique throughout the procedure. *Important:* Administer pain medication about 30 minutes before beginning the procedure, as ordered.

Position Mrs. Woodard flat on her back. Explain the procedure to her, and tell her why it's necessary. Then, position an emesis basin or bed-saver pad under the wound, to protect the bed linen.

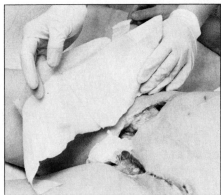

2 Put on nonsterile gloves. Remove the dressing from the wound, as shown here, and remove any previously-applied packing from the wound. (Earlier, this patient's packing was removed in a Hubbard tank.) Discard the soiled dressing in the plastic bag.

*Available in both the United States and in Canada

Wound management

Irrigating and packing a wound continued

3 Next, flush the wound with the mixture of hydrogen peroxide and saline solution. (As you see, this solution is bottled in a dark container, to protect the hydrogen peroxide from light.) Hold the solution bottle's tip about 2″ (5.1 cm) from the wound. Starting at the top of the wound (its cleanest portion), slowly squirt the solution into it. Continue to squirt solution into the wound, as you work toward the bottom (its least-clean portion). This removes loose debris and drainage from the wound. *Caution:* To avoid contaminating the bottle and solution, don't touch the wound with the top of the bottle, or aspirate solution back into the bottle.

▧ *Nursing tip:* If you prefer, use a bulb syringe to irrigate the wound. If the wound is small and deep, attach a soft rubber or latex catheter to the end of the syringe to facilitate irrigation.

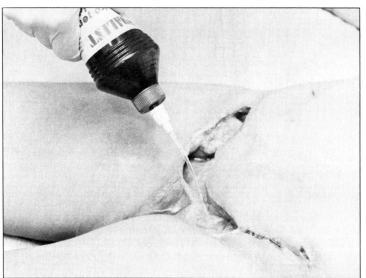

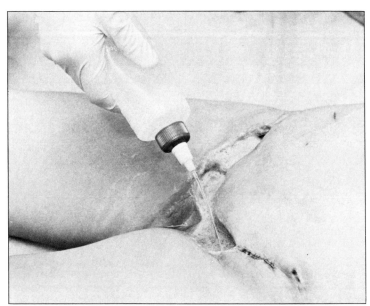

4 Now, rinse the wound with normal saline solution, using the same procedure described in step 3. Continue rinsing until the return fluid is clear (or as ordered). *Important:* Thoroughly rinse out the hydrogen peroxide solution before applying povidone-iodine.

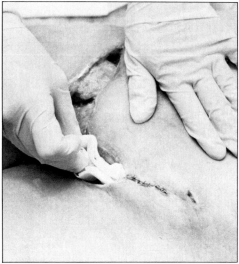

5 After you've finished irrigating and rinsing the wound, carefully pat it dry, using gauze pads. Again, work from the top of the wound to the bottom. Discard the pads in the plastic bag.

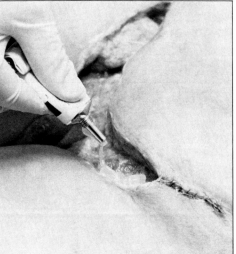

6 Uncap the tube of Elase ointment and squeeze a portion of it into the wound. As you know, this ointment helps debride the wound, and promotes healing from the inside.
Important: Don't let the tip of the ointment tube touch the wound.
Replace the cap on the tube.

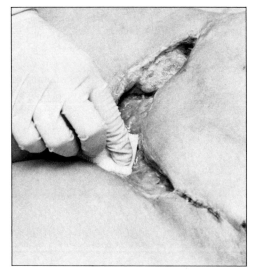

7 Spread a thin layer of Elase ointment around the inside of the wound, using a gauze pad. After you've finished, discard the pad in the plastic bag. Then, remove your gloves and discard them in the plastic bag, too.

8 Now you're ready to pack the wound. Place a roll of Kling gauze in the basin, taking care not to touch the gauze with your hands. Apply povidone-iodine solution, as shown here, until the roll's saturated.

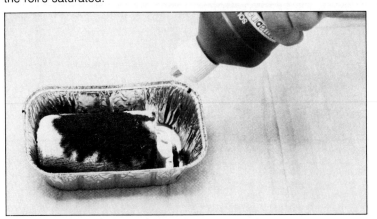

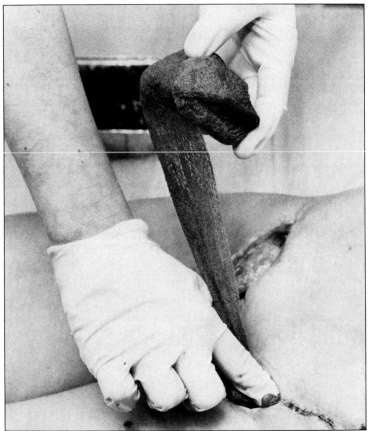

9 Put on a clean pair of gloves. Take the saturated roll of gauze and squeeze out excess solution. Pack it into the wound, unraveling the roll with one hand, and packing the gauze into the wound with the other. If necessary, use forceps to pack the gauze into the corners of a deep wound. *Note:* You'd pack a smaller wound with 4"x4" gauze pads. But always pack a large wound, like this one, with a continuous gauze roll. Gauze pads may become lost in a large wound.

10 Continue packing until the entire wound is filled, as shown. Then, cut off and discard any excess gauze.

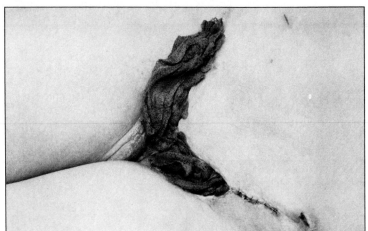

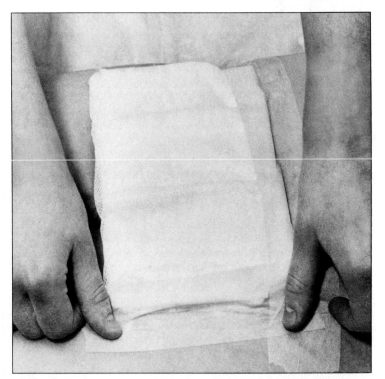

11 Remove your gloves and discard them in the plastic bag. Then, place a Surgipad over the packing, taking care not to touch its underside with your fingers. Tape the pad into place, as shown here. If your patient's ambulatory, consider applying a binder to provide security for the dressings. (For more on binders, see pages 136 and 137.)

Close the plastic bag with a fastener and discard it, according to your hospital's infection control standards. Wash and dry your hands.

Finally, document the procedure and your observations. Include the wound's appearance; the color, amount, consistency, and odor of any drainage; and the type of irrigating solution and packing you used.

Special considerations

Michael Feller just returned to your unit after having a Billroth II. You have a big responsibility. Besides caring for your patient's wound and the indwelling (Foley) catheter and naso-gastric tube he has in place, you'll also need to closely monitor his condition. Do you know what problems may threaten Mr. Feller's recovery?

Suppose, for example, he develops kidney failure. Can you recognize its earliest signs, and take appropriate action? And what if Mr. Feller goes into shock? Can you recognize shock's signs and symptoms? Do you know what action to take?

In this section, you'll find the answers to these questions. In addition, we'll tell you how to:
• identify common cardiovascular complications.
• recognize the signs of hypoxia.
• provide Foley catheter care.
• implement intermittent nasogastric suctioning.
• manage fluid and electrolyte imbalances.

Recognizing cardiovascular complications

Whenever you suspect a post-operative cardiovascular complication, be prepared to give your patient prompt, effective care. Begin by notifying the doctor. Then, reassure your patient and make him as comfortable as possible. Explain all procedures to him. Monitor him closely for signs and symptoms of shock, and start I.V. therapy, as ordered.

But, in addition to the above, what else should you do? That depends on the complication. The following chart will familiarize you with some common postoperative cardiovascular complications. Study it carefully.

Thrombophlebitis

Possible causes
• Prolonged bed rest
• Trauma
• Infection
• I.V. insertion; prolonged I.V. therapy
• Use of oral contraceptives

Signs and symptoms
• Heat, pain, swelling, redness, and induration along the length of the affected vein
• Swelling and cyanosis of affected arm or leg
• Malaise

Nursing interventions
• Instruct patient to avoid prolonged sitting or standing.
• Frequently inspect I.V. insertion sites for early signs of phlebitis, especially if large doses of drugs are administered I.V. If you observe any signs of phlebitis, remove the I.V. needle or catheter, and begin another I.V. in the opposite arm (if possible).
• Avoid using leg veins for I.V. therapy. Thrombophlebitis occurs more readily in long leg veins.
• Elevate affected arm or leg.
• Apply warm compresses to affected arm or leg.
• Offer analgesics, as ordered, to reduce pain.
• Administer anticoagulants, if ordered.
• Enforce bed rest during early stage of deep-vein thrombophlebitis.
• Once a day, measure and record the circumference of the affected arm or leg.
• Observe for signs of pulmonary embolism, especially if thrombophlebitis occurs in a deep leg vein. For information on pulmonary embolism, see pages 126 and 127.
Note: To prevent thrombophlebitis, encourage early ambulation and range-of-motion (ROM) exercises.

Hemorrhage

Possible causes
• Traumatic rupture or incision of a large blood vessel
• Arterial erosion, possibly caused by wound drain, wound packing, or sutures

Signs and symptoms
• Faintness and dizziness
• Rapid pulse
• Sweating
• Thirst
• Rapid, shallow respirations
• Slight increase in blood pressure in the very early stage, followed by a steady, possibly-fatal decrease
• Orthostatic hypotension

Nursing interventions
• Control the bleeding, if possible, by applying direct pressure to the wound. If you're unsuccessful, apply pressure to the proper pressure point.
• Stay with your patient, and calmly reassure him, while someone else notifies the doctor.
• Monitor vital signs every 5 to 10 minutes.
• Unless contraindicated, place the patient in Trendelenberg position to increase blood flow to brain. (If bleeding is from his head, position him flat on his back and elevate his legs instead.)
• Check to be sure you have blood available for transfusion. Initiate an emergency type and crossmatch, if necessary.
• Prepare the patient for a blood transfusion, as ordered.

Cerebrovascular accident

Possible causes
- Thrombosis
- Embolus
- Hemorrhage

Signs and symptoms
- Nausea and vomiting
- Partial to total paralysis
- Coordination loss
- Aphasia
- Headache
- Sensory impairment
- Incontinence
- Visual disturbances
- Hypertension
- Convulsions
- Coma

    Note: Onset of signs and symptoms may be either rapid, or slow and progressive (depending on cause).

Nursing interventions
- Make sure patient has open airway, and administer oxygen, as ordered.
- Remain with the patient and provide emotional support.
- Closely monitor patient's vital signs, and watch for signs of increasing intracranial pressure.
- To determine bleeding location, prepare patient for cerebral angiogram and/or lumbar puncture, if ordered.
- Avoid administering any narcotic drug, such as morphine sulfate*, because it may further depress your patient's respirations.
- Be alert for signs of myocardial infarction or atrial fibrillation.

Pulmonary edema

Possible causes
- Cardiac disease, including acute left ventricular failure, chronic heart failure, and mitral valve disease
- Circulatory overload
- Infection

Signs and symptoms
- Severe dyspnea, orthopnea, coughing
- Cyanosis, diaphoresis, tachycardia
- Pallor
- Widely-dispersed rales
- Frothy sputum (white or pink)
- S_3 or S_4 heart sounds
- Restlessness, fatigue

Nursing interventions
- Place patient in high Fowler's position and provide complete bed rest.
- Administer high-flow oxygen by face mask or nasal cannula, depending on arterial blood gas (ABG) measurements, as ordered.
- Insert an indwelling (Foley) catheter, as ordered, and record output every half hour.
- Attach patient to a cardiac monitor, or obtain frequent electrocardiograms (EKGs).
- Administer diuretics such as furosemide (Lasix*), I.V., as ordered.
- Be prepared to administer a fast-acting cardiac glycoside I.V., such as digoxin (Lanoxin*), lanatoside C (Cedilanid*), or ouabain, to increase cardiac output.
- Relieve agitation, and improve cardiac output by administering morphine sulfate*, if ordered.
- In severe cases, apply rotating tourniquets, if ordered.
- Remain with the patient throughout the acute phase, and provide emotional support.

Septicemia

Possible causes
- Break in aseptic technique during skin prep, or during surgery itself
- Introduction of microorganisms from any other invasive procedure; for example, I.V. therapy or Foley catheter insertion
- Break in aseptic technique during wound care, resulting in wound infection

Signs and symptoms
- Malaise
- Headache
- Chills, fever
- Abdominal distention
- Petechial or purpuric skin eruptions. Papular, pustular or vesicular lesions may also appear.

    Note: Onset may be sudden or gradual.

Nursing interventions
- Help doctor determine cause by obtaining cultures and sensitivity tests (blood, wound, and urine), as ordered.
- Administer antibiotics, as ordered.
- Frequently monitor vital signs and level of consciousness for signs of septic shock (see page 143).
- Be prepared to assist doctor in draining an infected wound.
- Be prepared to remove all invasive lines and insert new ones, using strict aseptic technique. Remember to send catheter tips to the laboratory for culturing.
- Carefully consider the patient's nutritional and fluid needs.

Cardiac arrest

Possible causes
- Circulatory collapse from vasodilation or hypovolemia
- Ventricular fibrillation from myocardial infarction, heart failure, anesthetics, electrical shock, electrolyte imbalance, ventricular irritation, or acute hemorrhage
- Ventricular standstill or asystole from hypoxia, acidosis, and/or hypercapnia, vagal stimulation, or hyperkalemia

Signs and symptoms
- Profound hypotension
- Profound bradycardia
- Seizure
- Loss of consciousness
- Cessation of respirations
- Absence of peripheral pulses or heart sounds

Nursing interventions
- Begin cardiopulmonary resuscitation (CPR) immediately.
- If arrest is caused by hemorrhage, stop bleeding (if possible) and provide large volumes of fluids I.V. until blood transfusions are available.
- Keep I.V. lines patent to ensure rapid drug administration. For patients with ventricular arrhythmias, keep lidocaine hydrochloride (Xylocaine*) at bedside for I.V. bolus administration.
- Frequently obtain arterial blood gas measurements. Watch for arrhythmias if the patient develops hypoxia, acidosis, or other metabolic abnormalities.
- Check for signs of cerebral edema and other central nervous system complications; for example, elevated temperature, widened pulse pressure, diminished level of consciousness, or seizure activity.
- Frequently monitor urinary output, urine's specific gravity, serum electrolytes, blood urea nitrogen (BUN), and creatinine levels. Administer an osmotic diuretic, if ordered, to increase urinary output and reduce risk of acute renal failure.
- Be alert for CPR complications such as cardiac tamponade or pneumothorax, caused by rib or sternal fractures.
- Closely monitor level of consciousness, skin color, peripheral pulses, and vital signs.
- Prepare patient for transfer to the ICU for monitoring of pulmonary artery pressure, cardiac output, and arterial blood pressure.

*Available in both the United States and in Canada

Special considerations

Learning about shock

Shock—whether hypovolemic, cardiogenic, septic, or neurogenic—is one of the most dangerous postoperative complications your patient may face. Can you recognize shock's earliest signs and symptoms? Doing so may save your patient's life.

To recognize shock, you must first understand how the circulatory system functions. As you probably know, adequate blood circulation depends on an equal balance of the following components: volume of circulating blood, vascular resistance, and effective cardiac output. When a profound imbalance of these components occurs—and the patient loses his ability to compensate—the circulatory system ceases to function properly. As a result, inadequate tissue perfusion may occur.

Inadequate tissue perfusion, which causes shock, leads to cell damage or death. The illustration below shows the cellular changes that occur when your patient develops shock.

The type of circulatory system imbalance determines the type of shock that develops. For example, decreased blood volume may lead to hypovolemic shock.

But, no matter what type of shock you're dealing with, the signs and symptoms are similar. Closely monitor your patient for:
• decreased temperature (except in early septic shock, when the patient's temperature may be elevated).
• tachycardia with weak, thready pulse.

• rapid, shallow respirations. In most types of shock, slow breathing appears late, after profound failure of the patient's compensatory mechanisms. In septic shock, however, the patient's respiration rate increases markedly as his condition worsens.
• hypotension with a narrowing of pulse pressure.
• cold, clammy skin (except in septic shock, when the patient's skin may feel warm and flushed).
• diminished urinary output (except in septic shock, which

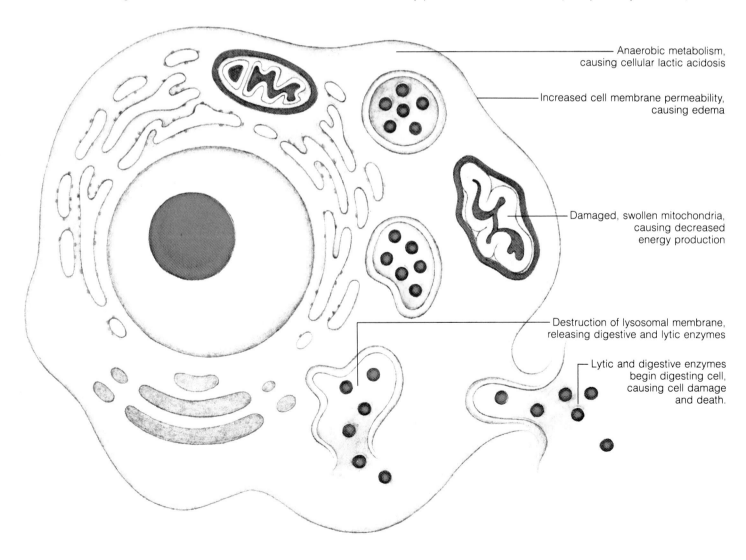

Anaerobic metabolism, causing cellular lactic acidosis

Increased cell membrane permeability, causing edema

Damaged, swollen mitochondria, causing decreased energy production

Destruction of lysosomal membrane, releasing digestive and lytic enzymes

Lytic and digestive enzymes begin digesting cell, causing cell damage and death.

may cause excessive urinary output).
• restlessness, confusion, anxiety. As shock deepens, the patient may become apathetic, delirious, or comatose.

Combating shock: Some guidelines

Do you know how to act on these signs and symptoms? The chart at right will give you specific instructions. Study it carefully. In addition, remember these guidelines that apply to all types of shock:
• Call the doctor immediately.
• Check to be sure patient has an open airway and adequate circulation. Start cardiopulmonary resuscitation (CPR), if necessary.
• Correct the cause of shock.
• Remain with the patient. Provide a calm, quiet atmosphere, if possible, and give emotional support.
• Record blood pressure, pulse rate, and other vital signs at least once every 15 minutes.
• Keep patient covered with a light blanket.
• Begin I.V. therapy, as ordered.
• Draw venous blood for type and crossmatch, complete blood cell count (CBC), and serum electrolytes, as ordered.
• Obtain arterial blood for arterial blood gas measurements. Treat any acid-base disturbances that may occur, as ordered.
• Assist doctor with insertion of central venous pressure (CVP) line for CVP readings and fluid replacement.
• Monitor intake and output. Insert an indwelling (Foley) catheter to measure urinary output, if ordered. If output is less than 30 ml/hour, carefully increase fluid infusion, as ordered, but be alert for signs of overhydration (see page 148).

Complication	Possible causes	Nursing interventions
Hypovolemic shock	Decreased blood volume resulting from blood loss, severe dehydration, third space sequestration (as in burns or pancreatitis), or abnormal fluid loss (for example, excessive vomiting or diarrhea)	• Place patient in Trendelenberg position, unless contraindicated. • Administer low-percentage oxygen. • To increase circulating blood volume, increase I.V. fluid rate until blood or blood products are available. Give volume expanders, such as albumin, if ordered.
Cardiogenic shock	Myocardial infarction, pericardial tamponade, cardiac arrest, or pulmonary artery embolism, resulting from stress of surgery and/or anesthesia	• Administer oxygen. • To improve cardiac output, administer an inotropic drug such as dopamine hydrochloride (Intropin*), I.V. drip, as ordered. • Place patient on cardiac monitor, or obtain an immediate electrocardiogram (EKG). • Make patient as comfortable as possible. • Prepare the patient for transfer to the intensive care unit (ICU). Prepare him emotionally for procedures he may undergo in the ICU; for example, pulmonary artery catheter insertion, or intra-aortic balloon pump insertion.
Septic shock Septic shock may produce these additional signs and symptoms: low-grade fever (except in burn patients who may be hypothermic), nausea, vomiting, abdominal cramps or distention, elevated white blood cell count, and increased blood urea nitrogen (BUN).	Cell destruction from endotoxins caused by a bacterial infection (usually gram negative)	• Make patient as comfortable as possible. • Obtain specimens for culture and sensitivity tests, as ordered. • Administer a broad-spectrum antibiotic, such as carbenicillin disodium (Pyopen*), as ordered. • If ordered, give patient a steroid, such as dexamethasone (Decadron*) to reduce inflammation and improve cardiovascular function. • Be prepared to transfer the patient to the ICU for continuous hemodynamic monitoring.
Neurogenic shock	Abnormal blood vessel dilation from cervical fracture, concussion, spinal cord injury, or spinal anesthetic	• Keep patient flat. • Be prepared to administer isoproterenol hydrochloride (Isuprel*), as ordered, to increase vascular resistance and elevate blood pressure. • Administer large volumes of fluid to correct hypovolemia.

*Available in both the United States and in Canada

Special considerations

Learning about hypoxia

Signs of hypoxia in a postoperative patient may signal a serious complication; for example, atelectasis, pneumonia, hypovolemic shock, or cardiac arrhythmias.

As you know, hypoxia is an oxygen deficiency in the patient's cell tissue, usually caused by an underlying disorder. Therefore, in addition to correcting the underlying disorder, treatment of hypoxia includes oxygen administration and assisted ventilation.

Since hypoxia can lead to tissue damage and death, make sure you know how to recognize its earliest signs and symptoms. Watch for:
• anxiety, restlessness, or disorientation
• rapid or irregular respirations
• wheezing, crowing, or gurgling sounds
• rhonchi or rales
• cyanosis or a rapid, thready pulse.

Identifying hypoxia's cause

Hypoxia can be caused by a number of underlying disorders. For example:
• A patient with a respiratory complication, such as atelectasis or pneumonia, may display signs of hypoxia because his alveoli are filled with secretions, preventing inspired oxygen from being exchanged through the alveoli walls into the bloodstream.
• If your patient has severe cardiac arrhythmias or pulmonary embolism, he may become hypoxic. The embolism or arrhythmias may block the absorption of oxygen into the bloodstream.
• Your patient may develop histotoxic hypoxia. In this condition, histotoxic chemicals produced by toxic wastes from invading microorganisms prevent oxygen from diffusing through cell walls. Chemicals, such as cyanide, may also have this effect on muscle and organ cells. To reverse histotoxic hypoxia, the causative microorganism must be identified as soon as possible and appropriate antibiotic therapy started.
• An anemic patient may also exhibit signs of hypoxia. Since oxygen binds to hemoglobin, any decrease in the patient's hemoglobin level will cause a decrease in his oxygen level. Check the patient's hematocrit and hemoglobin levels to determine if he's anemic. If so, your nursing care (as ordered) may include: administering oxygen, giving a blood transfusion for immediate relief of hypoxia, and helping the doctor determine the anemia's cause.
• Oxygen-affinity hypoxia is caused by specific disorders that affect blood; for example, hyperthermia, acidemia, or hypercapnia. These disorders change the bond between hemoglobin and oxygen. If the hemoglobin's ability to carry oxygen is decreased, your patient may show signs of hypoxia.

Important: Make sure you determine the underlying cause of hypoxia before giving oxygen to your patient. Because of its potency, oxygen may cause serious damage when used indiscriminately. For example, giving high concentrations of oxygen to a patient with chronic obstructive pulmonary disease (COPD) may actually reduce his respiratory rate; or, if your patient has a blocked upper airway, giving oxygen is useless because it can't reach his lungs.

Using intermittent nasogastric suction

1 *Elizabeth Kirby, a 58-year-old telephone operator, returns to your unit after a colectomy. She has a Levin-type single-lumen nasogastric (NG) tube in place. To prevent gastric distention and promote wound healing, the doctor orders long-term intermittent suction. Do you know how to proceed?*

If you're using a Gomco® Thermotic® Drainage Pump, familiarize yourself with it by examining this photo. To use it, take the steps detailed in this photostory.

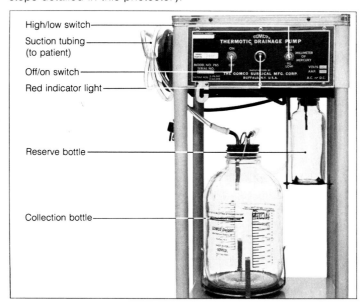

High/low switch
Suction tubing (to patient)
Off/on switch
Red indicator light
Reserve bottle
Collection bottle

2 Begin by explaining the procedure to Mrs. Kirby. Reassure her that suctioning won't be painful, and tell her why it's necessary.

For her comfort, place Mrs. Kirby in a semi-Fowler's position. Then, unpin the NG tube from her gown and check for correct tube placement. (For guidelines, see the NURSING PHOTOBOOK PERFORMING GI PROCEDURES.) When you're sure the tube's positioned correctly in the stomach, attach the NG tube connector to the suction tubing, as the nurse has done here.

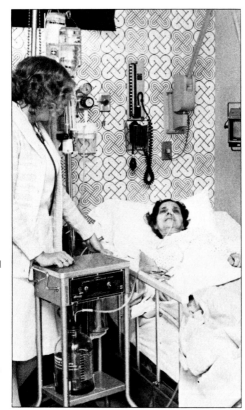

3 Next, set the suction machine for intermittent *low* suction, as shown. When used with a single-lumen NG tube like Mrs. Kirby's, intermittent *high* suction may damage her stomach wall and cause bleeding. You may use the high setting if your patient has a double-lumen NG tube (such as a Salem Sump®) in place and the doctor orders it.

Turn on the machine, and check to make sure it's functioning. If it is, the red indicator light in the middle of the front panel will blink continuously, at intervals of 10 to 20 seconds.

Document the time that you initiated suctioning.

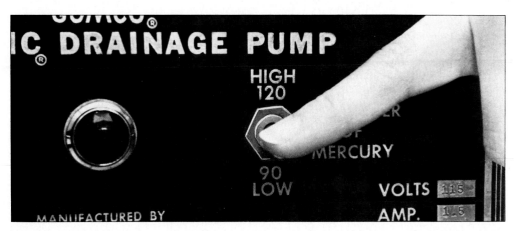

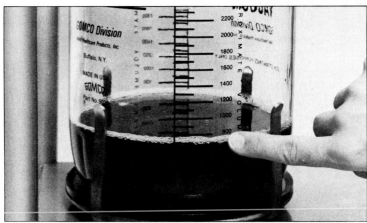

4 Throughout the treatment, periodically check your patient to make sure she's comfortable. To reduce throat discomfort caused by the NG tube, advise her to chew ice chips or hard candy (unless contraindicated).

Examine her nostril for any signs of erosion or a developing pressure sore. Make sure the tube's taped securely, and change the tape daily. (As an alternative, consider securing the tube with an NG tube holder. See page 120 of the NURSING PHOTOBOOK ENSURING INTENSIVE CARE.)

Also, observe the color of her gastric contents. The presence of blood may indicate stomach wall damage. (This is more likely to occur if the machine's set on high intermittent suction.) However, expect to see blood if your patient's recently undergone gastric surgery. Check the suction setting at least every 8 hours. (For guidelines on evaluating tube drainage, including drainage from an NG tube, see page 155 of this book.)

Also, check the equipment to make sure that proper suctioning is being maintained. Suspect loss of suctioning if your patient complains of nausea, or if you don't see gastric contents flowing periodically through the tubing and accumulating in the collection bottle.

🖂 *Nursing tip:* If your patient has a double-lumen NG tube in place, test for proper suctioning by holding the unattached lumen to your ear. A sucking noise confirms suctioning.

To correct loss of suctioning, check the rubber stoppers in the collection and reserve bottes. Fit them more tightly in the bottles, if necessary. Also, check all the tubing connections to make sure they're tight.

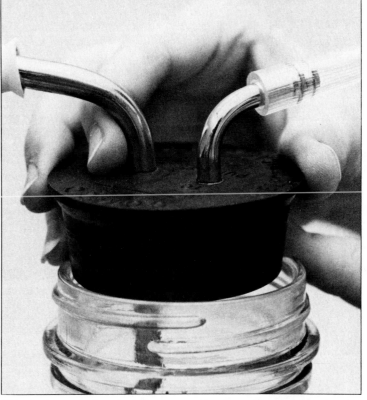

5 At the end of each shift, temporarily clamp the NG tube closed, and turn off the suction machine. Remove the collection bottle, and pour the contents into a measuring container. Rinse the collection bottle with warm tap water. Then, reconnect it, taking care to tightly fit the machine's rubber stopper into the bottle, as shown. (If necessary, follow the same procedure to empty, rinse, and reconnect the reserve bottle. However, proper monitoring of the equipment will usually prevent drainage from reaching the reserve bottle.) Unclamp the NG tube, and turn on the suction machine to resume treatment.

Measure all fluid collected, and document the amount and color in your nurses' notes and in the patient's intake and output record.

Finally, empty and rinse the measuring container and wash your hands.

Special considerations

Providing indwelling (Foley) catheter care

You know that urinary catheterization is a major cause of nosocomial infection. So, to avoid the need for catheterization, try these measures to help your postop patient urinate: place a warm compress over his bladder; pour warm water over his perineum; gently massage his suprapubic area; change his body position; or turn on the faucet in the bathroom—the sound of running water may be enough to help him urinate.

If these measures aren't successful, the doctor may then order catheterization. If he does, use strict aseptic technique when performing the procedure. Then, closely monitor your patient for these signs and symptoms of urinary tract infection: feelings of urgency, burning, and pain; concentrated, foul-smelling urine; pyuria, hematuria; or bleeding from the urinary meatus.

Important: If your patient develops a urinary tract infection,

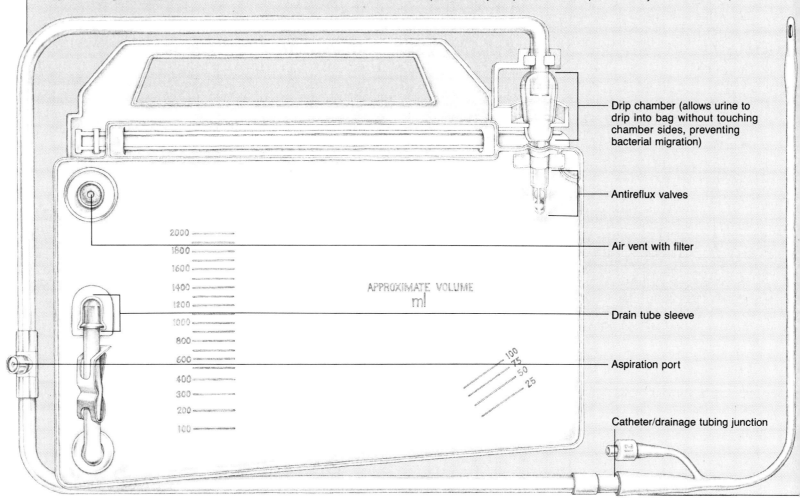

Drip chamber (allows urine to drip into bag without touching chamber sides, preventing bacterial migration)

Antireflux valves

Air vent with filter

Drain tube sleeve

Aspiration port

Catheter/drainage tubing junction

Assessing urine color

Straw-colored (dilute urine)	**Dark yellow or amber (concentrated urine)**	**Turbid or smoky**	**Red or red-brown**
Causes Nervous conditions, diabetes insipidus, granular kidney, large fluid intake	**Causes** Acute febrile diseases, low fluid intake, vomiting, diarrhea	**Causes** Blood, chyle, spermatozoa, prostatic fluid, fat droplets	**Causes** Porphyrin, hemoglobin, myoglobin, erythrocytes, transfusion reaction, hemorrhage, bleeding in urogenital tract, pyrvinium pamoate (Povan)

isolate him from patients who've recently returned from the OR. This precaution reduces the risk of cross-contamination.

If your patient returns from surgery with a Foley catheter in place—or if the doctor orders one for your patient after surgery—you'll have to take special precautions to help prevent a urinary tract infection and keep the catheter draining freely. Remember these important points:
• Wash your hands before and after touching the catheter, bag, or tubing.
• Check the catheter for proper drainage whenever you're caring for your patient.
• Don't allow the tubing to kink or loop, or it may block the urine flow, causing backflow into your patient's bladder. This may result in bladder distention and infection.
• Never clamp the drainage tubing, unless you're obtaining a urine specimen or transferring your patient. Then, clamp it only briefly.
• Keep the junction of the catheter and drainage tubing secured. If you must disconnect the tube from the catheter, use aseptic technique.
• Keep the bag below your patient's bladder level to permit drainage by gravity.
• Don't place the urine drainage bag on the floor, because the bag may become contaminated.
• Empty the drainage bag at least once every 8 hours, using strict aseptic technique.
• Never use the same measuring container (graduate) for more than one patient. This precaution significantly decreases the risk of cross-contamination.
• At least once daily, clean the urinary meatus. (If your patient's female, also clean her perineal area.) Examine the area for signs of irritation, infection, or erosion. When you do, avoid touching or moving the tubing.
• If the doctor orders a urinalysis or urine culture, obtain specimen through aspiration port only.
• If the catheter's obstructed, notify the doctor. Change the catheter only when ordered. (Remember, frequent catheter changes increase the risk of infection.)
• Provide adequate fluid intake to prevent residual urine pooling and possible infection.
• Administer fluids containing acid, such as cranberry juice, to acidify urine and inhibit microorganism growth.
• Document all procedures and observations.

Recognizing kidney failure

Surgery can have a traumatic effect on your patient's vital organs, particularly his kidneys. They may respond to surgical stress with partial or total shutdown.

Because of the potential for this complication, you must be able to recognize the signs and symptoms of kidney failure. Notify the doctor if you observe any of the following:
• change in quality and/or quantity of urine; for example, oliguria, anuria, or diluted or concentrated urine
• edema in dependent areas
• confusion and decreased level of consciousness
• hyperkalemia, hypermagnesemia, hypocalcemia, or metabolic acidosis, as indicated by lab test results.

The doctor may order the insertion of an indwelling (Foley) catheter for your patient if he hasn't urinated within 8 hours after surgery. *Important:* If you obtain less than 30 ml of urine per hour after inserting the catheter, notify the doctor.

If your patient develops kidney failure, take these precautions to avoid further complications:
• Remove the patient's Foley catheter (if present), if the doctor orders. This reduces the risk of urinary tract infection.
• Restrict all fluid intake to the amount ordered by the doctor.
• Measure urine output hourly if your patient still has a catheter in place; if he doesn't, take meticulous measurements whenever he urinates.
• Weigh your patient daily at approximately the same time. A good time is after he urinates, but before he eats. Always use the same scale, and make sure he wears the same (or similar) clothing.
• Collect blood and urine specimens for osmolality tests, if ordered.
• Frequently monitor blood urea nitrogen (BUN), creatinine, potassium, calcium, and magnesium levels in the blood.
• Avoid administering nephrotoxic drugs; for example, gentamicin sulfate (Garamycin*).
• Avoid administering drugs the liver doesn't detoxify (for example, potassium and some antacids). Otherwise, these drugs may accumulate to toxic levels in the bloodstream.
• Provide for your patient's nutritional needs. *Note:* The doctor may order that your patient's protein intake be reduced to prevent an increase in BUN levels.
• Carefully document all your findings.

Orange-red or orange-brown	Yellow-brown or green-brown	Dark brown, green-blue, or black	Cloudy white
Causes Drugs such as phenazopyridine hydrochloride (Pyridium*); urobilin	**Causes** Jaundice, obstruction of bile duct, phenol poisoning	**Causes** Methylene blue (MG-Blue), chorea, typhus	**Causes** Pus, blood, epithelial cells, fat, phosphate bacteria, colloidal particles, urates, all-vegetable diet

*Available in both the United States and in Canada

Special considerations

Nurses' guide to fluid and electrolyte imbalance

When you care for a patient who's had surgery, you expect fluid and electrolyte management to be challenging. On the one hand, your patient may lose fluid and electrolytes from wound bleeding and drainage. On the other hand, if he's received a general anesthetic, he may *retain* fluids and sodium. Why? Because general anesthetics can trigger production of antidiuretic hormone (ADH).

No wonder, then, that many postop patients experience fluid and electrolyte imbalance. Your goal is to provide your patient with enough fluid to maintain extracellular fluid and blood volume, without causing overhydration.

Learn how to identify and manage problems associated with fluid and electrolyte imbalances by reading the chart below. In addition, follow these guidelines whenever you suspect your

Problem	Causes	Signs and symptoms	Nursing considerations
Dehydration	• Inadequate fluid replacement during surgery • Excessive use of diuretics • Administration of osmotic agents (such as mannitol or dextrans) which may cause diuresis • Fever with excessive diaphoresis • Excessive gastrointestinal fluid losses from nasogastric drainage, diarrhea, or vomiting • Diuretic phase of renal disease	• Low-grade fever • Flushed skin, dry mucous membranes, poor skin turgor • Hypotension • Rapid pulse • Thirst • Muscle weakness • Oliguria • Elevated hematocrit and serum sodium levels • Weight loss	• Observe patient closely for insensible water loss from hyperventilation and diaphoresis. • Administer fluids, as ordered. *Important:* Assess the patient frequently during rapid administration of large volumes of fluid.
Overhydration	• Excessive ADH secretion • Administration of excessive fluids I.V.	• Weight gain • Muscle weakness • Moist rales; dyspnea • Increased blood pressure • Lethargy, apathy, disorientation • Edema in dependent body parts	• To prevent this condition, administer hypotonic solutions with caution. • To prevent this condition, especially in patients with cardiopulmonary disease, administer fluids cautiously (at specified rates). • Administer a diuretic, as ordered, if patient has received an excessive volume of fluids I.V.
Hypokalemia (serum potassium below 3.8 mEq/l)	• Potassium-free I.V. therapy (in a patient receiving nothing by mouth) • Excessive gastrointestinal fluid losses from nasogastric suctioning, vomiting, diarrhea, or intestinal fistula	• Possibly-fatal cardiac arrhythmias • Muscle weakness, fatigue, leg cramps • Anorexia, vomiting, paralytic ileus	• Obtain frequent electrocardiograms (EKGs). Observe for changes in heart rate, rhythm, and EKG pattern. • To correct the potassium imbalance, the doctor may order: increased potassium intake in diet, or oral potassium supplements (diluted to prevent irritation and to facilitate absorption); or, in emergency, slow administration of diluted potassium chloride I.V. (patient should be on cardiac monitor). • Monitor serum potassium level to determine effects of replacement therapy. • Determine source of potassium loss; for example, wound or fistula drainage. Analysis of the drainage sample's electrolyte content will help indicate amount of daily loss. • If patient's receiving digitalis, observe him for signs and symptoms of toxicosis. Hypokalemia can potentiate digitalis.

patient has an imbalance:
- Weigh the patient daily on the same scale. Make sure he's wearing the same (or similar) clothing each time.
- Maintain an accurate intake and output record, including all types of drainage; for example, blood, urine, cerebrospinal fluid, and vomitus.
- Closely monitor all laboratory test results. Immediately report

any change to the doctor.
- Observe the patient for specific signs and symptoms of fluid and electrolyte imbalance; for example, increased or decreased urine specific gravity, thirst, weight loss or gain, edema, poor skin turgor, or muscle weakness.

Note: For more details on fluid and electrolyte imbalance, see the NURSING PHOTOBOOK ENSURING INTENSIVE CARE.

Problem	Causes	Signs and symptoms	Nursing considerations
Hyperkalemia (serum potassium above 5.5 mEq/l)	• Excessive administration of potassium • Renal disease	• Cardiac disturbances including bradycardia, possibly-fatal arrhythmias, and cardiac arrest • Apathy, confusion • Areflexia, numbness, muscle weakness, tingling • Abdominal cramping, nausea	• Obtain frequent EKGs. Observe for changes in heart rate, rhythm, and EKG pattern. • Restrict ingestion of potassium. • Administer combination of glucose and insulin I.V., as ordered, to help shift potassium into cells. • As ordered, follow I.V. treatment with a potassium exchange resin, such as sodium polystyrene sulfonate (Kayexalate*); may be given orally, through nasogastric tube, or as an enema. During prolonged potassium-removal treatment, observe for signs of hypokalemia.
Hypocalcemia (serum calcium less than 8.9 mg/dl)	• Administration of large volumes of citrated stored blood. Citrate combines with calcium, preventing calcium utilization. • Cancer • Acute pancreatitis	• Muscle tremors, tetany, twitching • Cardiac arrhythmias • Anxiety, irritability	• Obtain frequent EKGs. Observe for changes in rate, rhythm, and pattern. • Monitor serum albumin level. Never give calcium gluconate or calcium chloride I.V. if serum albumin level is low. Hypercalcemia and arrhythmias may result. • If serum albumin level is normal, administer calcium gluconate or calcium chloride 10% I.V., as ordered. *Caution:* Administer slowly, to avoid causing arrhythmias.
Hyponatremia (serum sodium below 135 mEq/l)	*Hyponatremia associated with excess fluid:* • Inappropriate ADH syndrome • Excessive intake of hypotonic fluids during surgery *Hyponatremia associated with dehydration:* • Administration of diuretics • Excessive gastrointestinal fluid losses from nasogastric suctioning, vomiting, or diarrhea	*Hyponatremia associated with excess fluid:* • Headache • Anxiety, lassitude, apathy, confusion • Anorexia, nausea, vomiting, diarrhea, cramping • Hyperreflexia, muscle spasms, muscle weakness *Hyponatremia associated with dehydration:* • Irritability, tremors, seizure, coma • Dry mucous membranes • Low-grade fever • Hypotension, tachycardia • Decreased urine output ranging from oliguria to anuria	• Correct sodium and water imbalance through diet and administration of I.V. solutions; for example, 5% dextrose in normal saline solution, as ordered. • During administration of normal saline solution, observe patient closely for signs of hypervolemia (such as dyspnea, rales, and engorged neck or hand veins). • During treatments, monitor neurologic and gastrointestinal symptoms, to detect improvement or deterioration. • Monitor sodium and potassium levels closely.

*Available in both the United States and in Canada

Appendices

Analyzing a urine specimen

When your patient's urine specimen goes to the lab for analysis, do you know what happens to it? The lab technician will usually test it for characteristics and levels detailed in this chart. Notify the patient's surgeon and the anesthesiologist of any abnormal findings.

Characteristic	Normal finding	Abnormal findings	Possible causes
Color	Pale yellow to dark amber (varies with concentration)	• Colorless to straw-colored	• Excessive fluid intake • Chronic renal disease • Diabetes insipidus
		• Cloudy-white	• Parasitic disease
		• Yellow to amber with pinkish sediment	• Hyperuricemia and gout
		• Yellow to amber with whitish sediment	• Infection
		• Deep orange to orange-red	• Obstructive jaundice • Nonpathologic causes such as cascara sagrada, rhubarb, beets, senna
		• Orange-red or orange-brown to red	• Hemoglobinuria • Malaria • Internal bleeding • Porphyria • Nonpathologic causes such as Phenazopyridine hydrochloride (Pyridium*), phenolphthalein (Ex-Lax), phenolsulfonphthalein (PSP) dye
		• Green-blue or dark brown to black	• Melanoma • Nonpathologic causes such as methylene blue (MG-Blue)
Turbidity (lucidity)	Clear	• Cloudy	• Infection • Urinary tract disease • Nonpathologic causes such as presence of amorphous phosphate
Specific gravity (concentration as compared with H_2O)	1.010 to 1.025 (varies with hydration level)	• Dilute (1.001 to 1.010) or concentrated (1.025 to 1.030) urine	• Low specific gravity may be caused by renal disorders or diabetes insipidus. • Nonpathologic causes for high specific gravity include albumin, contrast media, or dextran.
Acidity (pH)	pH 4.8 to 7.5	• Greater than pH 7.5	• Renal acidosis • Calculi
Protein	Little to no protein	• Proteinuria	• Serious renal or proximal tubule disorder • Toxemia • Severe heart failure
Glucose	None	• Glycosuria	• Gestational diabetes • Diabetes mellitus • Nonpathologic causes such as dextrose therapy
Red blood cells	None to three per high-power field	• More than three per high-power field	• Renal malfunction or trauma to the urinary tract • Tumor or infection in the urinary tract
White blood cells	None to four per high-power field	• More than four per high-power field	• Bacterial infection
Casts	None	• Clear or yellowish, cylindrically-shaped cellular debris, visible under a microscope	• Renal damage

*Available in both the United States and in Canada

Interpreting a complete blood cell count (CBC)

Before your patient undergoes surgery, the doctor will order a routine complete blood cell count (CBC) for your patient. This test determines the number of blood components in relation to blood volume. In addition, it measures sedimentation rate.

As the following chart shows, the CBC distinguishes among several types of white blood cells (WBCs). These values are called the WBC differential.

To learn about normal CBC values, study the chart. You're responsible for informing the surgeon and anesthesiologist of any abnormal values, *before* the patient undergoes surgery. *Note:* CBC values considered normal may vary slightly from hospital to hospital, according to the testing methods used. Check your hospital's lab manual, or the information printed on the lab slip.

White blood cells (WBCs)
Normal values
4,100 to 10,900/microliter (µl)
Possible causes of abnormality
Above normal: Infection (such as an abscess, meningitis, appendicitis, or tonsillitis), leukemia, tissue necrosis (caused, for example, by burns, myocardial infarction, or gangrene), stress, allergy
Below normal: Viral infection (such as influenza, measles, infectious hepatitis, mononucleosis, or rubella), typhoid fever, bone marrow depression (caused, for example, by administration of antineoplastic drugs, ingestion of mercury or other heavy metals, or exposure to benzene or arsenic)

WBC differential
Normal values (percentage of total WBC count)
Neutrophils: 47.6% to 76.8%
Lymphocytes: 16.2% to 43%
Monocytes: 0.6% to 9.6%
Eosinophils: 0.3% to 7%
Basophils: 0.3% to 2%
Possible causes of abnormality
For detailed information, consult page 38 of DIAGNOSTICS in the NURSE'S REFERENCE LIBRARY™ Series.

Red blood cells (RBCs)
Normal values
Men: 4.5 to 6.2 million/µl
Women: 4.2 to 5.4 million/µl
Possible causes of abnormality
Above normal: Dehydration, polycythemia
Below normal: Hemorrhage, anemia from dietary deficiencies, sickle cell anemia, fluid overload

Hemoglobin
Normal values
Men: 14 to 18 g/dl (after age 40, 12.4 to 14.9 g/dl)
Women: 12 to 16 g/dl (after age 40, 11.7 to 13.8 g/dl)
Possible causes of abnormality
Above normal: Hemoconcentration (from polycythemia or dehydration)
Below normal: Anemia, pregnancy, recent hemorrhage, fluid retention (causing hemodilution)

Hematocrit
Normal values
Men: 42% to 54% of total blood volume
Women: 38% to 46% of total blood volume
Possible causes of abnormality
Above normal: Dehydration, polycythemia
Below normal: Anemia, acute hemorrhage, fluid overload

Platelets
Normal values
130,000 to 370,000/cu mm
Possible causes of abnormality
Above normal: Hemorrhage, hemoconcentration, pregnancy, inflammatory or infectious disorders, splenectomy, polycythemia, iron deficiency anemia

Below normal: Aplastic anemia, acute leukemia, thrombocytopenic purpura, administration of antineoplastic drugs, disseminated intravascular coagulation (DIC), infection

Erythrocyte sedimentation rate (ESR)
Normal values
Men: 0 to 10 mm/hour
Women: 0 to 20 mm/hour
Possible causes of abnormality
Above normal: Tissue destruction (either inflammatory or degenerative), pregnancy, menstruation, acute fever, cancer, infection, anemia
Below normal: Liver disease, polycythemia, sickle cell anemia, blood hyperviscosity, low serum protein

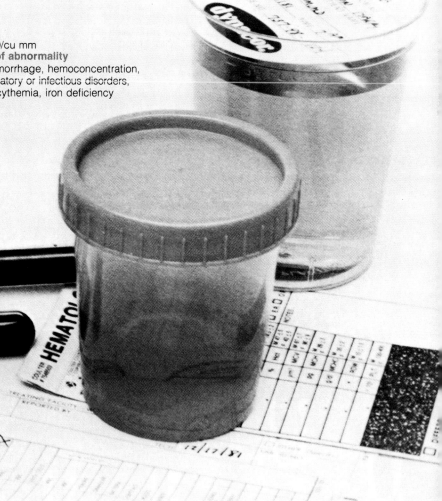

Appendices

Understanding routine blood studies

Before your patient undergoes surgery, the doctor will order blood serum analysis of some or all of the substances listed below. To perform this analysis, your hospital's laboratory may use an automated electronic system called the Sequential Multiple Analyzer (SMA®), or the Sequential Multiple Analyzer with Computer (SMAC®). These systems perform blood studies rapidly, economically, and comprehensively, and may identify unsuspected abnormalities.

In this chart, you'll find the normal levels for the most commonly-analyzed blood substances, and possible reasons for abnormal levels. However, keep in mind that levels considered normal may vary somewhat from hospital to hospital, depending on the specific testing methods used. Use the values from your hospital's laboratory manual.

Alkaline phosphatase

Normal range
Men: 90 to 239 units/l
Women under age 45: 76 to 196 units/l
Women over age 45: 87 to 250 units/l

Possible cause of abnormality
Above normal:
- Skeletal disease (rickets or osteomalacia)
- Hyperparathyroidism
- Mononucleosis
- Liver disease

Bilirubin, total

Normal range
0.1 to 1 mg/dl

Possible cause of abnormality
Above normal:
- Liver damage
- Pernicious anemia
- Eclampsia
- Biliary obstruction

Calcium

Normal range
8.9 to 10.1 mg/dl

Possible cause of abnormality
Above normal:
- Hyperparathyroidism
- Multiple myeloma
- Excessive ingestion of milk or antacids containing calcium
- Multiple fractures
- Prolonged bed rest
Below normal:
- Hypoparathyroidism
- Malnutrition
- Calcium malabsorption
- Renal failure
- Administration of large volumes of citrated, stored blood
- Acute pancreatitis

Carbon dioxide

Normal range
22 to 34 mEq/l

Possible cause of abnormality
Above normal:
- Respiratory acidosis
- Intestinal obstruction
- Vomiting, or continuous gastric drainage, causing metabolic alkalosis
- Primary aldosteronism
Below normal:
- Metabolic acidosis; for example, diabetic acidosis
- Renal failure
- Diarrhea, or continuous intestinal drainage
- Anesthesia, causing change in respiratory pattern

Cholesterol

Normal range
120 to 330 mg/dl

Possible cause of abnormality
Above normal:
- Nephrotic syndrome
- Bile duct blockage
- Hypothyroidism
- Pancreatitis
- Lipemia
- Excessive cholesterol in diet
Below normal:
- Malnutrition
- Pernicious and hemolytic anemia
- Hyperthyroidism

Creatinine

Normal range
Men: 0.8 to 1.2 mg/dl
Women: 0.6 to 0.9 mg/dl

Possible cause of abnormality
Above normal:
- Destruction of more than 50% of the kidney's nephrons
- Acromegaly
- Gigantism

Albumin

Normal range
3.5 to 5 g/dl

Possible cause of abnormality
Above normal:
- Multiple myeloma
Below normal:
- Liver or renal disease
- Hodgkin's disease
- Peptic ulcer
- Malnutrition
- Plasma loss from burns
- Diarrhea
- Acute cholecystitis
- Collagen disease
- Hyperthyroidism

Blood urea nitrogen (BUN)

Normal range
8 to 20 mg/dl

Possible cause of abnormality
Above normal:
- Mercury poisoning
- Obstructive uropathy
- Renal disease
- Excessive protein in diet
- Digestion of blood from gastrointestinal (GI) tract bleeding
Below normal:
- Severe hepatic damage
- Malnutrition
- Overhydration

Chloride

Normal range
100 to 108 mEq/l

Possible cause of abnormality
Above normal:
- Severe dehydration
- Renal failure
- Primary aldosteronism
- Head injury (causing neurogenic hyperventilation)
Below normal:
- Prolonged vomiting
- Gastric suctioning
- Addison's disease
- Excessive use of diuretics

Glucose (fasting)

Normal range
80 to 120 mg/dl

Possible cause of abnormality
Above normal:
- Diabetes mellitus
- Pancreatitis
- Hepatic disease
- Anoxia
- Strenuous exercise
- Convulsive disorders
- Administration of excessive glucose I.V.
Below normal:
- Hyperinsulinism
- Insulinoma
- Hepatic insufficiency
- Addison's disease
- Hypoglycemia

Lactic dehydrogenase (LDH)	Serum glutamic-oxaloacetic transaminase (SGOT)
Normal range 100 to 225 mU (milliunits) per ml	**Normal range** 8 to 20 units/l
Possible cause of abnormality *Above normal:* • Pulmonary infarction • Liver disease • Shock • Myocardial infarction • Renal, brain, or skeletal muscle damage • Pernicious, hemolytic, or sickle cell anemia • Muscular dystrophy • Blood specimen hemolysis	**Possible cause of abnormality** *Above normal:* • Hepatitis • Cholecystitis • Myocardial infarction • Mononucleosis
Potassium	**Sodium**
Normal range 3.8 to 5.5 mEq/l	**Normal range** 135 to 145 mEq/l
Possible cause of abnormality *Above normal:* • Renal failure • Addison's disease • Blood specimen hemolysis • Tissue breakdown or hemolysis from injury • Excessive administration of potassium supplements *Below normal:* • Excessive use of diuretics • Cushing's syndrome	**Possible cause of abnormality** *Above normal:* • Dehydration • Pyloric obstruction • Administration of hypertonic saline solution *Below normal:* • Excessive use of diuretics • Vomiting • Diarrhea • Diaphoresis • Gastrointestinal suctioning • Inadequate sodium intake • Adrenal insufficiency
Protein, total	**Uric acid**
Normal range 6.6 to 7.9 g/dl	**Normal range** Men: 4.3 to 8 mg/dl Women: 2.3 to 6 mg/dl
Possible cause of abnormality *Above normal:* • Dehydration • Diabetic acidosis • Chronic infection • Multiple myeloma • Monocytic leukemia • Shock *Below normal:* • Hemorrhage • Malnutrition • Hodgkin's disease • Blood dyscrasia • Eclampsia • Hypertension • Severe burns	**Possible cause of abnormality** *Above normal:* • Gout • Leukemia • Impaired renal function • Toxemia of pregnancy *Below normal:* • Defective reabsorption of uric acid by kidney tubules, possibly from shock • Acute hepatic atrophy

Understanding preop EKGs

A preop electrocardiogram (EKG) is usually routine for any patient older than 35. You're responsible for making sure the patient's doctors know about any cardiac arrhythmias the EKG reveals. To learn more about them, read this chart.

Sinus bradycardia
• 60 beats per minute (BPM) or less

Description
• Regular rhythm
• Normal waveform configuration and electrical conduction

Possible causes
• Increased intracranial pressure
• Vagal stimulation
• Sick sinus syndrome
• Treatment with beta-blockers and sympatholytic drugs
Important: Sinus bradycardia may be normal in an athlete.

Sinus tachycardia

Description
• 100 to 180 BPM
• Regular rhythm
• Normal waveform configuration and electrical conduction

Possible causes
• Congestive heart failure
• Myocardial infarction
• Anemia
• Pulmonary embolism
• Sympathomimetic drugs
Note: Sinus tachycardia may be a normal response to fever, preop anxiety, or pain.

Premature atrial contractions (PACs)

Description
• Variable rate
• Irregular rhythm, due to premature P waves
• P waves may be inverted or irregularly-shaped
• P wave may appear or may be buried in the preceding T wave
• P-R intervals may be extended because of premature P waves
• QRS complexes follow P waves, except in blocked PACs
• QRS complex usually normal

Possible causes
• Vagal stimulation
• Congestive heart failure
• Rheumatic valvular disease
• Electrolyte imbalance
• Ischemic heart disease
• Cor pulmonale
• Acute respiratory failure
• Atrial disease or enlargement
• Chronic obstructive pulmonary disease
• Treatment with digitalis, aminophylline, or sympathomimetic drugs
• Anxiety
• Excessive caffeine consumption

Atrial flutter

Description
• Atrial rate from 250 to 350 BPM; ventricular rate variable
• Atrial rhythm regular; ventricular rhythm variable
• P waves have saw-tooth shape
• QRS complexes uniform in shape; may be irregular in rate

Possible causes
• Congestive heart failure
• Coronary artery disease
• Valvular heart disease (such as rheumatic heart disease)
• Myocardial infarction
• Pulmonary embolism
• Hypertension

Atrial fibrillation

Description
• Atrial rate 350 to 600 BPM; ventricular rate variable
• Irregular rhythm
• P waves absent
• P-R intervals can't be measured
• QRS complexes uniform in shape, but irregular in rate
• Rapid fibrillation may cause a nearly-straight waveform

Possible causes
• Coronary artery disease
• Rheumatic heart disease
• Hypertension
• Pericarditis
• Pulmonary embolism
• Mitral stenosis
• Cardiomyopathy
• Myocardial infarction
Note: Patients with chronic atrial fibrillation are very prone to postop pulmonary embolism.

Appendices

Understanding preop EKGs continued

Premature ventricular contractions (PVCs)

Description
- Variable rate; QRS complex premature and usually followed by a complete compensatory pause after PVC
- QRS complex wide and distorted; QRS complex usually premature in relation to prevailing rhythm
- S-T segment and T wave usually in opposite direction of QRS complex
Note: PVCs can occur singly, in pairs, or in groups of three or more. They may alternate with normal beats, and are considered most ominous when clustered and multifocal with R wave on T pattern.

Possible causes
- Coronary artery disease
- Congestive heart failure
- Myocardial infarction
- Cardiomyopathy
- Hypoxia
- Drug toxicosis (possibly caused by digitalis, aminophylline, tricyclic antidepressants, or beta-adrenergics)
- Hypokalemia
- Stress
- Hypercalcemia
- Rheumatic heart disease
- Hypertension
- Excessive caffeine consumption

Ventricular tachycardia (VT)

Description
- Ventricular rate 100 to 270 BPM; atrial rate variable
- Regular atrial rhythm; ventricular rhythm may be regular or irregular
- P wave normal when visible
- P wave relationship to QRS complex variable
- QRS complexes wide, bizarre, and independent of P waves

Possible causes
- Myocardial infarction, myocardial ischemia, or ventricular aneurysm
- Digitalis or quinidine toxicosis
- Hypokalemia or hyperkalemia
- Hypercalcemia
Note: Some patients may have short runs of ventricular tachycardia without being symptomatic.

First degree AV block

Description
- Variable rate (usually 60 to 100 BPM)
- Regular rhythm
- P waves normal
- P-R interval prolonged (greater than 0.2 seconds)
- QRS complex normal

Possible causes
- Inferior or anterior wall myocardial infarction or ischemia
- Digitalis, quinidine, or procainamide hydrochloride toxicity
- Hyperkalemia
- Rheumatic heart disease, causing conduction pathway scarring
Note: Some anesthetics may cause further prolongation of P-R interval, which could lead to other life-threatening arrhythmias.

Second degree AV block (Wenckebach or Mobitz Type I)

Description
- Variable heart rate (atrial rate greater than ventricular rate)
- Irregular ventricular rhythm; regular atrial rhythm
- P-R interval becomes progressively longer with each consecutive cycle until QRS complex disappears (dropped beat). After a dropped beat, P-R interval shortens; then becomes gradually longer until another beat is dropped.
- P waves precede QRS complex, but QRS complex may not follow each P wave
- QRS complex usually normal

Possible causes
- Inferior wall myocardial infarction
- Digitalis, quinidine, or procainamide hydrochloride toxicosis
- Vagal stimulation
- Rheumatic heart disease
Note: If your patient has this type of heart block, the doctor will probably postpone surgery.

Second degree AV block (Mobitz Type II)

Description
- Variable heart rate (atrial rate greater than ventricular rate)
- P-R interval usually normal, consistent with QRS complex
- QRS complex may not follow each P wave
- Ventricular rhythm may be irregular with pause caused by missing QRS complex. (Two identical P-R intervals precede a dropped QRS complex.)
- QRS complex usually wide, with bundle branch configuration

Possible causes
- Degenerative disease of conduction system
- Ischemia of AV node caused by anterior myocardial infarction
- Digitalis toxicosis
Note: If your patient has this type of heart block, the doctor will probably cancel surgery.

Third degree AV block (complete heart block)

Description
- Regular atrial rate; slow, regular ventricular rate (usually 20 to 45 BPM)
- Atrial and ventricular rates and rhythms are independent of each other
- No constant P-R interval
- Appearance of QRS complex may be normal (junctional pacemaker), or wide and bizarre (ventricular pacemaker)

Possible causes
- Digitalis toxicosis
- Myocarditis
- Cardiomyopathy
- Myocardial infarction or ischemia
- Hypoxia
Note: Consider this an emergency. Notify the doctor as soon as you see the results. He may insert a pacemaker.

Acknowledgements

Assessing drainage from tubes and catheters

After major surgery, most patients have a drainage tube or catheter in place. Do you know how much drainage you can expect to see from drainage tubes and catheters, and how to evaluate its color, odor, and consistency? Use this chart as a guide.

Drainage system	Type of drainage	Daily amount	Color	Odor	Consistency
Indwelling (Foley) catheter	Urine	1,000 to 2,500 ml	Clear, yellow	Ammonia	Watery
Gastrostomy tube	Gastric contents	Up to 1,500 ml	Pale, yellowish-green	Sour	Watery
Surgical evacuator	Wound drainage	Varies with procedure; from 500 to 1,000 ml initially (from hip surgery, for example), to as little as 5 ml for a small wound	Varies with procedure; usually sanguineous to serosan-guineous	Like wound dressing	Variable; from thick, clotted blood to serous (watery) fluid
Ileal conduit	Urine	500 to 2,500 ml	Clear, yellow	Ammonia	Watery (with mucus and blood initially)
Ileostomy	Small bowel contents	Up to 4,000 ml in first 24 hours; then, less than 500 ml	Brown	Sour, fecal	Initially serous with mucus; brown liquid stool when peristalsis resumes
Miller-Abbott tube	Intestinal contents	Up to 3,000 ml	Dark green or brown	Neutralized acid, fecal	Thick
Nasogastric tube	Gastric contents	Up to 1,500 ml	Pale, yellowish-green	Sour	Watery
T tube	Bile	500 ml	Bright yellow to dark green	Acrid	Thick
Suprapubic catheter	Urine	500 to 2,500 ml	Clear, yellow	Ammonia	Watery
Ureteral catheter	Urine	250 to 1,250 ml	Clear, yellow	Ammonia	Watery

We'd like to thank the following people and companies for their help with this PHOTOBOOK:

ACME UNITED CORPORATION
Medical Products Division
Bridgeport, Conn.
James F. Farrington
Senior Vice President, Marketing

ALLIED HEALTHCARE PRODUCTS, INC.
Gomco Division
St. Louis, Mo.

AMERICAN HAMILTON
Division American Hospital Supply Corp.
Two Rivers, Wis.

BARD-PARKER
Division Becton, Dickinson and Co.
Lincoln Park, N.J.

W. A. BAUM CO., INC.
Copiague, N.Y.

CHESEBROUGH-POND'S INC.
Hospital Products Division
Greenwich, Conn.

CODMAN & SHURTLEFF, INC.
Randolph, Mass.

DAVOL, INC.
Subsidiary of C.R. Bard, Inc.
Cranston, R.I.

HOSPITAL MARKETING SERVICES CO., INC.
Naugatuck, Conn.

THE JOBST INSTITUTE, INC.
Toledo, Ohio

JOHNSON & JOHNSON PRODUCTS INC.
Patient Care Division
New Brunswick, N.J.

THE KENDALL COMPANY
Boston, Mass.

J.T. POSEY CO.
Arcadia, Calif.

PURITAN-BENNETT CORPORATION
Bellmawr, N.J.

J. SKLAR MFG. CO., INC.
Long Island City, N.Y.

SNYDER LABORATORIES, INC.
New Philadelphia, Ohio

SPARTA INSTRUMENT CORPORATION
Hayward, Calif.
Karen Ann Hubitsky, Product Manager

WELCH ALLYN, INC.
Skaneateles Falls, N.Y.
Douglas Hufnagle, Advertising Manager

Ivan L. Roth
University of Georgia
Athens, Ga.

Also the staffs of:

CHESTNUT HILL HOSPITAL
Philadelphia, Pa.

COMMUNITY GENERAL HOSPITAL
Reading, Pa.

HOSPITAL OF THE UNIVERSITY OF PENNSYLVANIA
Philadelphia, Pa.

QUAKERTOWN HOSPITAL
Quakertown, Pa.

THOMAS JEFFERSON UNIVERSITY HOSPITAL
Department of Radiology
Philadelphia, Pa.
George H. McArdle
Technical Administrator

Selected references

Books

Abels, Linda F. MOSBY'S MANUAL OF CRITICAL CARE: PRACTICES AND PROCEDURES, NINETEEN SEVENTY-NINE. St. Louis: C.V. Mosby Co., 1979.

Artz, Curtis P., and James D. Hardy, eds. MANAGEMENT OF SURGICAL COMPLICATIONS, 3rd ed. Philadelphia: W.B. Saunders Co., 1975.

Bordicks, Katherine J. PATTERNS OF SHOCK: IMPLICATIONS FOR NURSING CARE, 2nd ed. New York: Macmillan Pub. Co., Inc., 1980.

Brunner, Lillian S. THE LIPPINCOTT MANUAL OF NURSING PRACTICE, 2nd ed. Philadelphia: J.B. Lippincott Co., 1978.

Brunner, Lillian S., and Doris S. Suddarth. TEXTBOOK OF MEDICAL-SURGICAL NURSING, 4th ed. Philadelphia: J.B. Lippincott Co., 1980.

CONTROLLING INFECTION. Nursing Photobook™ Series. Springhouse, Pa.: Springhouse Corporation, 1981.

COPING WITH NEUROLOGIC DISORDERS. Nursing Photobook™ Series. Springhouse, Pa.: Springhouse Corporation, 1981.

Given, Barbara A., and Sandra J. Simmons. GASTROENTEROLOGY IN CLINICAL NURSING, 3rd ed. St. Louis: C.V. Mosby Co., 1979.

GIVING CARDIAC CARE. Nursing Photobook™ Series. Springhouse, Pa.: Springhouse Corporation, 1981.

Holloway, Nancy M. NURSING THE CRITICALLY ILL ADULT. Reading, Mass.: Addison-Wesley Pub. Co., 1979.

IMPLEMENTING UROLOGIC PROCEDURES. Nursing Photobook™ Series. Springhouse, Pa.: Springhouse Corporation, 1981.

Kozier, Barbara B., and Glenora L. Erb. FUNDAMENTALS OF NURSING: CONCEPTS AND PROCEDURES. Reading, Mass: Addison-Wesley Pub. Co., 1979.

LeMaitre, George D., and Janet A. Finnegan. THE PATIENT IN SURGERY: A GUIDE FOR NURSES, 4th ed. Philadelphia: W.B. Saunders Co., 1980.

Luckmann, Joan, and Karen C. Sorenson. MEDICAL-SURGICAL NURSING: A PSYCHOPHYSIOLOGIC APPROACH, 2nd ed. Philadelphia: W.B. Saunders Co., 1980.

Massachusetts General Hospital. MASSACHUSETTS GENERAL HOSPITAL DEPARTMENT OF NURSING OPERATING ROOM PROCEDURE MANUAL. Reston, Va.: Reston Pub. Co., 1981.

Metheny, Norma M., and W.D. Snively. NURSES' HANDBOOK OF FLUID BALANCE, 3rd ed. Philadelphia: J.B. Lippincott Co., 1979.

Montag, Mildred L., and Alice R. Rines. HANDBOOK OF FUNDAMENTAL NURSING TECHNIQUES. New York: John Wiley and Sons, Inc., 1976.

NURSING DRUG HANDBOOK™. Nursing82 Books. Springhouse, Pa.: Springhouse Corporation, 1981.

PERFORMING GI PROCEDURES. Nursing Photobook™ Series. Springhouse, Pa.: Springhouse Corporation, 1981.

Phipps, Wilma J., et al. MEDICAL-SURGICAL NURSING: CONCEPTS AND CLINICAL PRACTICE. St. Louis: C.V. Mosby Co., 1979.

PROVIDING EARLY MOBILITY. Nursing Photobook™ Series. Springhouse, Pa.: Springhouse Corporation, 1980.

PROVIDING RESPIRATORY CARE. Nursing Photobook™ Series. Springhouse, Pa.: Springhouse Corporation, 1979.

Robinson, Corinne J., and Marilyn R. Lawler. NORMAL AND THERAPEUTIC NUTRITION, 15th ed. New York: Macmillan Pub. Co., Inc., 1977.

Rodman, Morton J., and Dorothy W. Smith. CLINICAL PHARMACOLOGY IN NURSING. Philadelphia: J.B. Lippincott Co., 1974.

Rosoff, Arnold J. INFORMED CONSENT. Rockville, Md.: Aspen Systems Corp., 1980.

Rossman, Isadore, ed. CLINICAL GERIATRICS, 2nd ed. Philadelphia: J.B. Lippincott Co., 1979.

Sabiston, David C., Jr., ed. DAVIS-CHRISTOPHER TEXTBOOK OF SURGERY, 11th ed. Philadelphia: W.B. Saunders Co., 1977.

Sutton, Audrey L. BEDSIDE NURSING TECHNIQUES IN MEDICINE AND SURGERY, 2nd ed. Philadelphia: W.B. Saunders Co., 1969.

Thompson, Martha. SHOCK SYNDROME: MECHANISMS AND MANIFESTATIONS; NURSING ASSESSMENT INTERVENTION AND EVALUATION. Reading, Mass.: Addison-Wesley Pub. Co., 1978.

Tilkian, Sarko M., et al. CLINICAL IMPLICATIONS OF LABORATORY TESTS, NINETEEN SEVENTY-NINE, 2nd ed. St. Louis: C.V. Mosby Co., 1979.

Williams, Sue R. ESSENTIALS OF NUTRITION AND DIET THERAPY, 2nd ed. St. Louis: C.V. Mosby Co., 1978.

Periodicals

Croushore, Theresa M. *Postoperative Assessment: The Key to Avoiding the Most Common Nursing Mistakes,* NURSING79, 9:46-51, April 1979.

DeSimone, Donna, et al. *Postoperative Complications—How to Help the Patient When Everything Goes Wrong,* NURSING81, 11:50-53, March 1981.

Dossey, B., and J.M. Passons. *Pulmonary Embolism: Preventing It, Treating It,* NURSING81, 11:26-33, March 1981.

Finn, Kathleen L. *How's Your Post-op Ambulation Technique?* RN, 42:69-72, September 1979.

Fry, E.N.S. *Postoperative Analgesia,* NURSING TIMES, 73:655-656, May 5, 1977.

Haines, Janice. *Anesthesia Part 1,* JOURNAL OF PRACTICAL NURSING, 29:14-19, November 1979.

Jackson, B.S., and P.M. Carlisle. *How Post-op Complications can Burgeon Into Crisis,* RN, 44:26-32, January 1981.

Juliani, Louise. *Assessing Renal Function,* NURSING78, 8:34-35, January 1978.

Lyons, Mary Lou. *What Priority Do You Give Preop Teaching?* NURSING77, 7:12-14, January 1977.

McConnell, Edwina A. *After Surgery: How You Can Avert the Obvious Hazards...and the Not-So-Obvious Ones, Too,* NURSING77, 7:32-39, March 1977.

McConnell, Edwina A. *Toward Complication-Free Recoveries For Your Surgical Patients, Part 1,* RN, 43:30-33, June 1980.

McConnell, Edwina A. *Toward Complication-Free Recoveries For Your Surgical Patients, Part 2,* RN, 43:34-38, July 1980.

Marcinek, Margaret Boyle. *Stress in the Surgical Patient,* AMERICAN JOURNAL OF NURSING, 77:1809-1811, November 1977.

Risser, Nancy L. *Preoperative and Postoperative Care to Prevent Pulmonary Complications,* HEART AND LUNG, 9:57-68, January-February 1980.

Roberts, Sharon L. *Renal Assessment: A Nursing Point of View,* HEART AND LUNG, 8:105-113, January-February 1979.

Schrankel, Dawn P. *Pre-operative Teaching,* SUPERVISOR NURSE, 9:82-90, May 1978.

Smith, B.J. *Safeguarding Your Patient After Anesthesia,* NURSING78, 8:52-56, October 1978.

Steele, Bonnie G. *Test Your Knowledge of Postoperative Pain Management,* NURSING80, 10:76-78, March 1980.

Weaver, Terri E. *New Life for Lungs...Through Incentive Spirometry,* NURSING81, 11:54-58, February 1981.

West, B. Anne. *Understanding Endorphins: Our Natural Pain Relief System,* NURSING81, 11:50-53, February 1981.

Index

Index